SpringerBriefs in Population Studies

Population Studies of Japan

The world population is expected to expand by 39.4 % to 9.6 billion in 2060 (UN World Population Prospects, revised 2010). Meanwhile, Japan is expected to see its population contract by nearly one-third to 86.7 million, and its proportion of the elderly (65 years of age and over) will account for no less than 39.9 % (National Institute of Population and Social Security Research in Japan, Population Projections for Japan 2012). Japan has entered the post-demographic transitional phase and will be the fastest shrinking country in the world, followed by former Eastern bloc nations, leading other Asian countries that are experiencing drastic changes.

A declining population that is rapidly aging impacts a country's economic growth, labor market, pensions, taxation, health care, and housing. The social structure and geographical distribution in the country will drastically change, and short-term as well as long-term solutions for economic and social consequences of this trend will be required

This series aims to draw attention to Japan's entering the post-demographic transition phase and to present cutting-edge research in Japanese population studies. It will include compact monographs under the editorial supervision of the Population Association of Japan (PAJ).

The PAJ was established in 1948 and organizes researchers with a wide range of interests in population studies of Japan. The major fields are (1) population structure and aging; (2) migration, urbanization, and distribution; (3) fertility; (4) mortality and morbidity; (5) nuptiality, family, and households; (6) labor force and unemployment; (7) population projection and population policy (including family planning); and (8) historical demography. Since 1978, the PAJ has been publishing the academic journal *Jinkogaku Kenkyu* (The Journal of Population Studies), in which most of the articles are written in Japanese.

Thus, the scope of this series spans the entire field of population issues in Japan, impacts on socioeconomic change, and implications for policy measures. It includes population aging, fertility and family formation, household structures, population health, mortality, human geography and regional population, and comparative studies with other countries.

This series will be of great interest to a wide range of researchers in other countries confronting a post-demographic transition stage, demographers, population geographers, sociologists, economists, political scientists, health researchers, and practitioners across a broad spectrum of social sciences.

More information about this series at http://www.springer.com/series/13101

Shuichirou Ike

Fertility Decline and Background Independence

Applying a Reaction-Diffusion System as a Stochastic Process

Springer

Shuichirou Ike
Department of Sociology
Teikyo University
Hachioji, Tokyo
Japan

ISSN 2211-3215 ISSN 2211-3223 (electronic)
SpringerBriefs in Population Studies
ISSN 2198-2724 ISSN 2198-2732 (electronic)
Population Studies of Japan
ISBN 978-4-431-55150-8 ISBN 978-4-431-55151-5 (eBook)
DOI 10.1007/978-4-431-55151-5

Library of Congress Control Number: 2015945157

Springer Tokyo Heidelberg New York Dordrecht London

Printed on acid-free paper

Springer Japan KK is part of Springer Science+Business Media (www.springer.com)

I dedicate this monograph to my devoted partner Takako with love.

Preface

The decline of fertility that was evident in Europe in the nineteenth century was not caused by industrialization. Fertility decline occurred in southwestern France as a unique and independent reaction-diffusion process and this process proceeded in parallel with industrialization as a whole.

The independence of the phenomenon of fertility decline from the prevailing socioeconomic conditions has been positively demonstrated by diffusionist scholars such as Coale, Knodel, and van de Walle. (See *The Decline of Fertility in Europe* [15].)

The absence of a causal relation between fertility decline and industrialization was astounding. Further pursuit of this remarkable occurrence would have led to the discovery of previously unexamined laws of sociology, in which demography involved.

However, since the emergence of household economics, this amazing phenomenon has been completely forgotten. Academic knowledge has not developed in a linear manner; it evidently retreated a considerable extent. Household economics has yielded no novel findings. It is only suggestive.

We may assume that the fertility decline resulted from a stochastic process, with the number of children born to each set of parents primarily attributed to the influence of residential neighbors on the parents in terms of their choices regarding the desired number of children. We can then provide reasonable explanations relating to key aspects of fertility decline such as *irreversibility, stability, and smoothing*. Moreover, we can specify the geographical location and historical period of the initial perturbation toward fertility decline. This space-time point is named a singularity of fertility decline in this book. We can further estimate the location and time of onset of a singularity of fertility decline by means of the velocity of a progressive (or traveling) wave.

Tokyo
June 2015

Shuichirou Ike

Acknowledgments

It is a pleasure for me to express my gratitude to Prof. Toshihiko Hara, who introduced me to this publication. I admire his considerable efforts to disseminate the findings of Japanese demographic studies.

I am also grateful for the efforts of Mr. Hirati of Springer Japan, who has worked with me on this publication.

I respectfully express my appreciation to the programmers who design and maintain important software such as Linux, LaTeX, Mendix, Gnuplot, and Octave.

In developing this study, I am indebted to the early diffusionists. Without the insights gained from their preceding studies, I could not have conceived of the reaction-diffusion equation. The integral equation that I have proposed for marriage function is solidly grounded in the work of A.J. Coale and G. Hernes.

Contents

List of Figures

List of Tables

Acronyms

DESDC	Difference Equation of the Spatial Distribution of Children
GSS	General Social Survey
JGSS	Japanese General Social Survey
MFDDE	Macro Fertility Decline Difference Equation
NDISD	Neighborhood-Dependent Isotropic Stochastic Decision
NFR	National Family Research
RDE	Reaction-Diffusion Equation
SDSMF	Space-Dependent Stochastic Marriage Function
SSM	Social Stratification and Mobility

Chapter 1
Background Independence of Fertility Decline

Abstract The theoretical framework of demographic transition that has been applied to explain fertility decline has failed completely. This has been evident since the 1980s, with the emergence of the diffusionist scholars. Reflecting on the achievements of these researchers, I employ Japanese case studies that exemplify the absence of a causal relationship between fertility decline and the processes of industrialization, urbanization, popularization of education, as well as mortality decline. In other words, I show that fertility decline is a stochastic diffusion process that is independent from its background context. We can observe several decisive phenomena that are characteristic of the diffusion process in Europe and Japan. Once we accept the fallacy of demographic transition and, instead, adopt the diffusion hypothesis, we can clearly grasp the fact that the explanation of fertility decline provided by household economics is not even wrong as I explain in the following chapter.

Keywords Fertility decline · Demographic transition · Diffusion hypothesis · Background independence

Ever since the industrial revolution and the emergence of classical economics, or Auguste Comte's formulation of the stage theory of development, we have considered socioeconomic alterations to be the primary and most powerful factor that changes human behaviors. A typical example of the stage theory of development within demography is the demographic transition theory. However, in light of empirical evidence of its numerous contradictions, this theory has now been debunked.

First, the stage theory of development is an illusion of modernity. In fact, the "modern" is itself an illusion. It is merely an intuition and not a scientific theory. This is because it cannot produce any falsifiable predictions. In fact, we are unable to understand the mechanism of any kind of alteration of society. We have not found any regularities or law-like processes in the development of society. The underlying reason for this failure is that we have commonly assumed that alterations in society can be attributed to human subjectivity and active changes resulting from socioeconomic alterations.

This common assumption does not lead us to the regularities we seek. In fact, there are profound regularities to be found in unsuspected places. I suggest that demographic phenomena have a distinctive property, namely, autonomy. From the

S. Ike, *Fertility Decline and Background Independence*,
Population Studies of Japan, DOI 10.1007/978-4-431-55151-5_1

time of the emergence of the diffusion hypothesis propounded by A.J. Coale and others [15] in 1986, it has been manifestly clear that fertility decline in Europe cannot be attributed to socioeconomic factors.

During the same period, the hypothesis formulated within household economics, and in the absence of positive data, dazzled many with its superficial generality. According to this hypothesis, it is implicitly and explicitly assumed that the interests of parents change as a result of socioeconomic developments. This assumption is commonplace and, therefore, almost false because its validity solely depends on human subjective reflection. Human subjective reflection cannot be the base of scientific inference.

Moreover, fertility decline is not related to socioeconomic developments. We should conceive of fertility behaviors as being independent from economic development. The Japanese pension system is in danger of collapsing owing to the low fertility rate of the Japanese. China embarked on an astonishing path of economic development by means of implementing a one child policy, and, for the same reason, is heading equally as fast toward ruin.

Demographic transition theory is grounded on the thesis that socioeconomic developments alter people's behaviors. Hereafter, I refer to this thesis as "background dependence." I will show that this thesis has been disproven, and will introduce in its place, an antithetical concept, that I refer to as "background independence" of fertility decline.

1.1 The Fallacies of Demographic Transition Theory

1.1.1 A Decline of Mortality Is not the Cause of a Decline of Fertility

Demographic transition theory suggests that a decline of mortality is the cause of fertility decline. Specifically, it posits that parents experience redundancy in relation to the number of their children. This subjective feeling then causes them to adhere to Malthusianism. However, this simplistic explanation can be empirically negated.

The first country that experienced fertility decline was France. Prior to the nineteenth century, fertility had already begun to decline in the country. At that time, however, there was no decline in the death rate in France. (see Table 1.1). Around 1800, the infant mortality rate was still high in France. Notwithstanding this high infant mortality rate, French couples had already begun having fewer children. It is clear that fertility decline began during a period of high mortality levels.

Table 1.1 shows that fertility began to decline in Germany and Hungary despite very high infant mortality rates in these countries. At the onset of the decline of fertility, infant mortality rates diverged widely. These data are evidence of the independence of fertility decline from mortality, which is one aspect of the background context.

Table 1.1 Demographic and socioeconomic indexes at onset of fertility decline for selected countries

	Date of decline in martial fertility by 10 %	Marital fertility before decline (I_g)	Index of proportion married (I_m)	Overall fertility (I_f)	Infant mortality per thousand	Percent of male labor force in agriculture	Percent rural[d]	Percent in cities over 20,000 population	Percent Illiterate[e]
France	ca. 1800	0.70	0.51[a]	0.30	185[c]	70	81	7	High
Belgium	1882	0.82	0.44	0.35	161	30	56	22	0.30
Switzerland	1885	0.72	0.44	0.29	165	33	78	9	Low
Germany	1890	0.76	0.50	0.39	221	38	68	21	Low
Hungary	ca. 1890	0.63	0.70	0.45	250	73	84	11	49[f]
England and Wales	1892	0.68	0.48	0.31	149	15	28	57	Low
Sweden	1892	0.71	0.42	0.31	102	49	81	11	Low
Scotland	1894	0.75	0.42	0.31	124	13	27	49	Low
Netherlands	1897	0.85	0.45	0.35	135[c]	29	26	42	Low
Denmark	1900	0.68	0.47	0.32	131	42	61	23	Low
Norway	1904	0.75	0.42	0.30	76	37	72	18	Low
Austria	1908	0.68	0.51	0.36	205	40	–	19	21
Finland	1910	0.70	0.46	0.31	114	66	85	9	44
Italy	1911	0.68	0.54	0.36	146	46	38	28	39
Bulgaria	1912	ca. 0.70	ca. 0.74	ca. 0.45	159	70	82	7	60

(continued)

Table 1.1 (continued)

	Date of decline in martial fertility by 10 %	Marital fertility before decline (I_g)	Index of proportion married (I_m)	Overall fertility (I_f)	Infant mortality per thousand	Percent of male labor force in agriculture	Percent rural[d]	Percent in cities over 20,000 population	Percent Illiterate[e]
Spain	1918	0.64	0.51	0.30	158	66	45	26	46
Ireland	1929	0.71	0.35	0.23	69	48	73	20	Low
Costa Rica	1962	0.89[b]	0.50[b]	0.57	74	58	66	20	14
Taiwan	1963	0.70	0.70	0.42	49	47	42	31	30
Chile	1964	0.65[b]	0.50[b]	0.39	103	37	29	53	15
Thailand	ca. 1970	ca. 0.75	0.75	ca. 0.51	77	75	85	12	18

Notes country borders are of the date of decline. All figures refer to the year estimated as the date of a 10 % decline in marital fertility except the index of the level of marital fertility before decline. Estimates were obtained by interpolation or extrapolation when data were not directly available for the year indicated

[a]In 1831

[b]Excluding consensual unions

[c]Children dead after registration only

[d]In communities of fewer than 5,000 or legal definition

[e]Both sexes, aged 10+ or 15+; high refers to percentages of young adults unable to sign their name on the marriage certificate or of illiterate army recruits, exceeding 50 %; low refers to percentages under 10 %

[f]6+

Source adapted with additions and correlations from Etienne van de Walle and Jhohn Knodel, "Demographic transition and fertility decline: The European case," *Contributed papers: Sydney Conference, International Union for the Scientific Study of Population*, 1965, p. 55

J. Knodel and Etienne van de Walle [36], pp. 221–222

Table 1.2 Order of the onset of the infant mortality and marital fertility declines

Country	Numbers of units	Infant mortality declines first	Marital fertility (I_g) declines first	Both at the same time
Switzerland	181	172	8	1
Germany	71	36	34	1
Belgium	9	1	8	–

Source Francine van de Walle, Infant Mortality and Demographic Transition [15], p. 228

1.1.1.1 Consistencies and Inconsistencies

Demographic transition theory assumes that fertility decline occurs as a response of sets of couples to a decline of mortality. If this assumption is correct, a decline of mortality must precede a decline of fertility. However, there are many evident exceptions that counter this assumption.

Table 1.2 shows that in nearly half of the counties in Germany, fertility began to decline before infant mortality declined. In Belgium, eight out of nine counties experienced marital fertility decline before a decline of infant mortality occurred. This shows that the assumption that fertility decline occurs as a response of sets of couples to a decline of mortality is undeniably false.

These inconsistencies relating to the order of the onset of infant mortality and marital fertility require a new theory of fertility decline for their explanation. Diffusion theory meets this requirement.

1.1.2 Industrialization

Table 1.1 shows that England and Wales lagged considerably behind France, Belgium, and Switzerland in terms of fertility decline. Thus, the most advanced industrial country at that time was not the first country to experience fertility decline (Figs. 1.1, 1.2 and 1.3).

Figure 1.4 shows that there was no decline of fertility in England and Wales in 1870. A decline of fertility had not yet begun in Birmingham, Liverpool, Manchester, and Greater London, which were all highly industrialized according to the prevailing standards.

In contrast to England and Wales, France began to experience fertility decline at the end of the eighteenth century. It is generally accepted that the industrialization process in France began after the Napoleonic Wars. In other words, fertility decline in France bore no relation with industrialization.

> Indeed, the first country to show signs of fertility decline was France, where birth rates started to fall around the time of the French Revolution. France could hardly be considered very advanced at the time in terms of any standard definition of development.
>
> J. Knodel and van de Walle [36], p. 224.

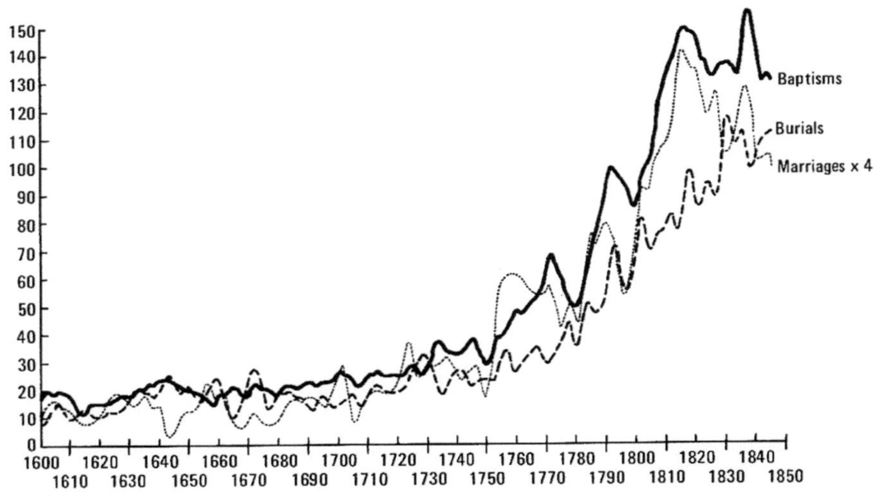

Fig. 1.1 Baptisms, burials, and marriages in Shepshed. **Source* D. Levine [46], p. 59

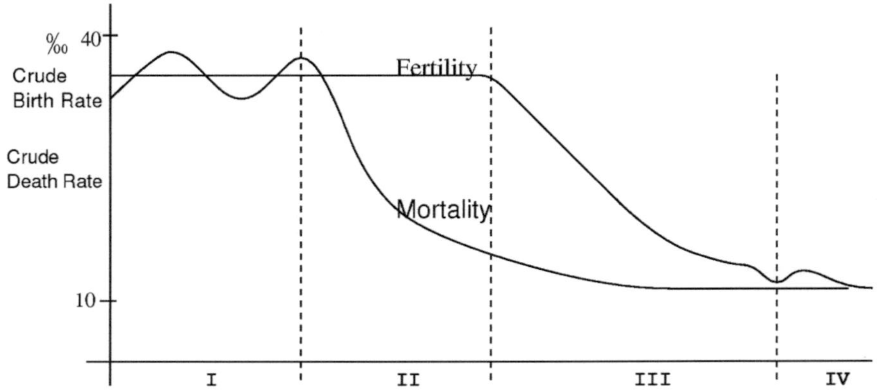

Fig. 1.2 Changes in fertility and mortality according to demographic transition theory

We can, thus, definitively conclude that industrialization was not the cause of fertility decline in France.

1.1.2.1 Lack of Concrete Causality

How could industrialization lead to a decline in the number of children for each set of parents? Household economists argue that the value of children changes. To adjust to changes brought about by industrialization, each set of parents would change the value they impute to children. The question that arises is whether this is a falsifiable hypothesis. I will subsequently critique this hypothesis in the Sect. 1.3. In brief, there are real arguments to refute it.

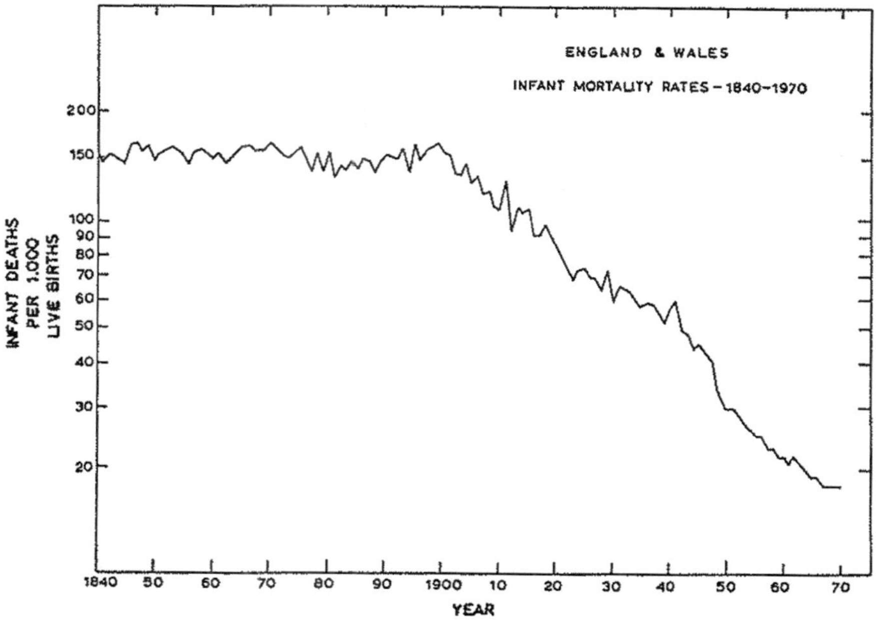

Fig. 1.3 Change in the infant mortality rate in England and Wales. *Source* M.W. Beaver [1], p. 244

One study has shown that during the process of industrialization, Shepshed, an England village, evidenced an increase in the number of children of each set of parents. This impressive study, conducted by D. Levine [46], mainly applied the family reconstruction method. From 1740 to 1840, baptisms, burials, and marriages demonstrated a positive correlation. Economic development in Shepshed brought about an increase in marriages. Moreover, there was no reduction in the number of children for each set of parents. Thus, the value of children did not change. Throughout the nineteenth century, child labor within English families exceeded that of present day families in Asia and Africa. As noted by Bertrand Russell, "Napoleon was defeated by English children and Russian mud".

As Table 1.3 shows, there was a decline in the survival rates of infants and children from 1600 to 1844. During the period of the Industrial Revolution, there was a reduction in e^0 (expected life span at birth). Increasing the number of their children was a reasonable response on the part of each set of parents in these circumstances. However, this differs unequivocally from the assumed relation between fertility and industrialization within demographic transition theory.

Industrialization does not necessarily lead to a decline of mortality. In the absence of industrialization, fertility declined in France. We cannot, therefore, find any concrete causal relation between industrialization and fertility decline. It is impossible to find a reasonable explanation of how industrialization resulted in a change in the value of children.

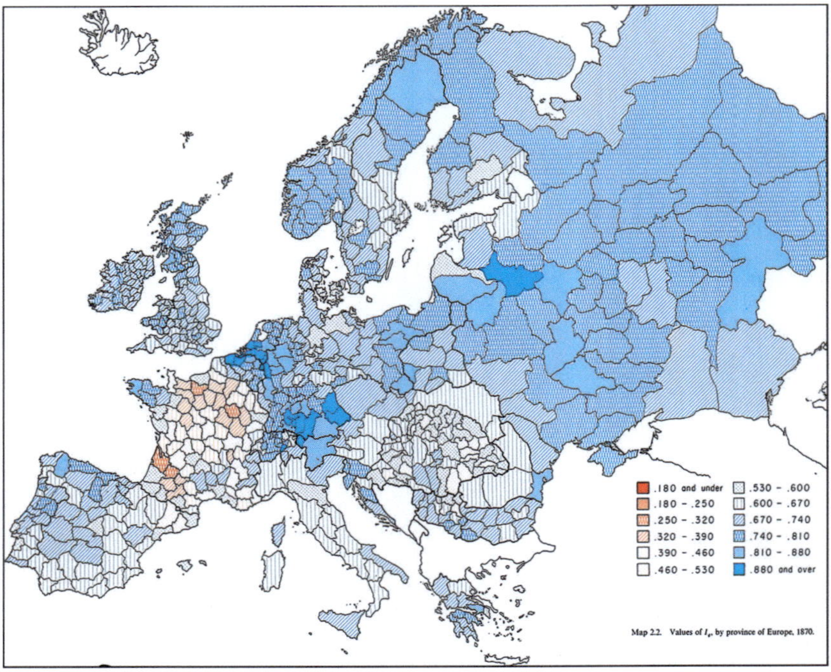

Fig. 1.4 Map 2.2. Values of I_g by province in Europe, 1870. *From here to the captions are the same as the original

1.1.3 Urbanization

Returning to Table 1.1, it is evident that there is no uniformity in the relations between fertility decline and urbanization. At the end of the eighteenth century, France was still not completely urbanized. In particular the southwestern part of France, where fertility decline is thought to have first started, was not entirely urbanized. In England and Wales, where urbanization was the most advanced, fertility decline began in the latter half of the nineteenth century, at the earliest. This counter evidence is exactly deniable. The early diffusionists also held this view as the following excerpt shows.

> Industrialization dose not even necessarily occur first in urban places. No one expects the same combination of factors to create industrialization in each country. Why should fertility decline be any different? Thus, urbanization or urban-rural differentials may or may not play a role in determining or explaining the onset of a decline in fertility. For example, we could examine whether rapid urbanization precedes fertility decline. France and England clearly present two different cases. The goal of finding a general explanation for the timing of this fertility decline in Europe was probably an illusory quest.
>
> Allan Sharin [60], p. 258.

There is another reason why urbanization cannot be regarded as the cause of a decline of fertility. This centers on the question of what urbanization actually is. We cannot provide an accurate scientific definition for it. Thus, while we intend, somehow, to understand what it is, we are not able to precisely define it. It is a misconception that we can explain fertility decline by employing this ambiguous concept. The attempt to explain fertility decline by employing the concept of industrialization may be criticued for the same reason.

1.1.4 Education

Education is commonly postulated to play a role in demographic transition. However, the question of why educated couples decrease the number of children they have remains. There is no reasonable causal explanation for this. Does the value of children change for educated couples? Did this actually occur?

Table 1.3 Infant and child mortality (MF) of shepshed

Cohort	Reconstitution					Ledermann		
	Age	At risk	Dying	Rate per thousand	Survivors	e^0	Rate per thousand	Survivors
1600–1699	0–1	1531	194	126	1000	49.18	126	1000
	1–4	1104	82	74	874		80	874
	5–9	788	26	33	809		24	804
	10–14	577	9	16	782		15	785
					770			772
1700–1749	0–1	1254	194	155	1000	44.02	158	1000
	1–4	905	85	94	845		96	842
	5–9	645	21	33	766		28	761
	10–14	493	6	12	741		17	740
					732			727
1750–1824	0–1	4096	639	158	1000	44.02	158	1000
	1–4	2977	281	94	842		96	842
	5–9	1953	65	33	763		28	761
	10–14	1342	26	19	738		17	740
					724			727
1825–1849	0–1	832	173	208	1000	37.05	207	1000
	1–4	415	63	152	792		162	793
	5–9	188	13	69	672		41	665
	10–14	64	1	16	625		26	638
					615			621

D. Levine. *Family Formation in an Age of Nascent Capitalism* quoted from [46], p. 68, Table 5.7
e^0 is expected life span at birth
*Ledermann is the life table selected by S. Ledermann from the Princeton "regional" model life table

1.1.4.1 Educated but with Many Children

We somehow believe that educated couples have fewer children than those who are poorly educated. However, this is an illusory perception, because the effect of marriage duration is not considered when making this comparison. There are many instances of highly educated individuals who had many children. Some examples follow.

Soseki Natume

Soseki Natsume was a famous Japanese novelist. He enrolled in Tokyo University in 1890. In 1900, the Japanese government sent him to Great Britain for further studies. Natsume was one of the most highly educated individuals in Japan at that time. In spite of his pessimism expressed in his novels, he had two sons and five daughters.

Charles de Gaulle

Born in 1890, de Gaulle was the third of five children. His father, Henri de Gaulle, was a professor of history and literature at a Jesuit College, who eventually founded his own school (http://en.wikipedia.org/wiki/Charles_de_Gaulle). Thus, despite being highly educated, the parents of Charles de Gaulle had five children.

de Gaulle's birth in 1890 in Nord Départment in the north of France, near the border with Belgium is especially noteworthy. The profound significance of this will become apparent in chapter two. It should also be noted that the number of children in the de Gaulle family was higher than the average number of children per family in France at that time. An average of 2.67 children was recorded for French women within the 1866–1875 cohort, who had completed their fertility (source: P. Festy [24]).

Ludwig Josef Johann Wittgenstein

Born in Vienna in 1889, Ludwig Josef Johann Wittgenstein was the last of eight children born to his parents. His father was one of the richest members of the European bourgeoisie, and his mother was an accomplished pianist. Although they were highly educated for their time, his parents had eight children in all.

Eight children per family was common in Austria at the end of nineteenth century. It is, therefore, reasonable to infer that there was no relation between education, belonging to the bourgeoisie, or being highly educated and the number of children born to each set of parents.

Ronald Aylmer Fisher

Born in 1890, Ronald Aylmer Fisher had two sons and six daughters. The man who defined the F-distribution did not change the value he assigned to children. His erudition and extraordinary genius in the field of applied mathematics did not lead him to think that the quality of children who were born was more important than the number of children born. Even though the number of children born to his neighbors declined, he had more children than the average couple for that period.

Fisher himself was the seventh of eight children born to his parents. His father was at one time a successful auctioneer and fine arts dealer.

Acquiring the highest level of education did not prevent him from having eight children. Rather, his obsession about the knowledge of population genetics and social Darwinism reinforced his will to produce more children.

Education has no Effect on Fertility

We can find no consistent trend in the relation between education and fertility. Contrary to common belief, education has no effect on fertility. There are several questions to consider. Is the objective of education to train by spending a lot of money on each child's education? Is the purpose of education to be a utilitarian or elitist? Did the fertility of the Europeans decline because they were educated according to one or the other of these objectives? If so, education is highly problematic. However, I believe that the social functions of education are more neutral. Education did not and does not change human nature.

1.1.4.2 Japanese Public Education

In 1905, more than 90 % of Japan's population had undergone an elementary education (see Table 1.4). It is estimated that fertility decline in Japan began between 1910 and 1920.

If elementary education had in fact resulted in a change in the value of children, Japan's fertility decline should have started from the nineteenth century when elementary education was prevalent. This shows that elementary education bears no relation to fertility decline. Public elementary education did not lead to a change in the value of children in Japan.

This leads to the next question relating to secondary and higher education, which is addressed in Table 1.5.

Fertility decline in Japan is evidently associated with the prevalence of secondary and higher education (see Table 1.6). An increase in the ratios of individuals with a secondary and higher educational background was associated with a decline of fertility in Japan.

Table 1.4 The number of primary schools and changes in the education attendance rate

	The number of primary school	Attendance rate		
		All	Male	Female
1875	20,017	35.4	50.8	18.7
1880	28,410	41.1	58.7	21.9
1885	28,283	49.6	65.8	32.1
1890	26,017	48.9	65.1	31.1
1895	26,631	61.2	76.7	43.9
1900	26,857	81.5	90.6	71.7
1905	27,407	95.6	97.7	93.3
1910	25,910	98.1	98.8	97.4
1915	25,578	98.5	98.9	98.0
1920	25,639	99.0	99.2	98.8
1925	25,459	99.4	99.5	99.4
1930	26,637	99.5	99.5	99.5

Note the attendance rate (percent) is the ratio to all of the children
Source The Ministry of Education (Japan), *History of Japanese Education System: Data Book "GakuseiHyakunensi"*
Table 1.1 made from pp. 214–215
http://www.mext.go.jp/b_menu/hakusho/html/others/detail/1317930.htm

Table 1.5 Changes in the secondary education attendance rate in Japan

Age at 1960	Cohort year	Year at age 15	The ratio of whose educational background is secondary (%)		
			All	Male	Female
35–39	(1921–1925)	(1936–1940)	32.7	34.4	30.6
40–44	(1916–1920)	(1931–1935)	27.0	29.4	25.2
45–49	(1911–1915)	(1926–1930)	25.6	28.3	23.2
50–54	(1906–1910)	(1921–1925)	21.9	24.3	19.6
55–59	(1901–1905)	(1916–1920)	16.1	19.2	13.3
60–64	(1896–1900)	(1911–1915)	12.9	15.6	10.2

Source Statistic Bureau of Japan, *Population of Japan*, 1960, Tokyo, Table 52, pp. 296–497
Hiroshi Kawabe [33], pp. 3–4

1.1.4.3 Mere Quasi Correlations

These associations could be considered as mere quasi correlations, because the sets of parents with an elementary educational background also evidenced a reduction in their fertility alongside their further education background. Almost all parents who only had an elementary educational background were peasants. They had no reason to have fewer children. Farming was not mechanized in Japan, and therefore they needed their families to serve as a work force. Those who accept the revealed

Table 1.6 Children of each set of parents by the husband's education attainment

Age at 1960	Born year	Year at age 20	Means of ever born			
			All	Primary	Secondary	Higher
35–39	(1921–1925)	(1941–1945)	2.86	3.04	2.54	2.28
40–44	(1916–1920)	(1936–1940)	3.50	3.67	3.13	2.84
45–49	(1911–1915)	(1931–1935)	4.18	4.37	3.70	3.37
50–54	(1906–1910)	(1926–1930)	4.68	4.90	4.01	3.56
55–59	(1901–1905)	(1921–1925)	4.93	5.12	4.08	3.55
60–64	(1896–1900)	(1916–1920)	4.97	5.12	4.16	3.63

Source Statistic Bureau of Japan, *1960 Population Census 10% sample Series 3 (Fertility)*, Tokyo, 1964, Table 1.2, pp. 174–175.
Hiroshi Kawabe [33], p. 6

preference hypothesis would argue that elementary education did change the value of children. Nonetheless, when they had a clear economic advantage in that they had a rational reason not to bear fewer children, they reduced their fertility.

What actually is the value of children? No one can define this concretely and precisely. The value of children is not a scientifically defined variable. Rather, it is merely subjective and suggestive. Science cannot be built on such a fragile base. Because of this lack of scientific objectivity, the hypothesis put forward within household economics is a theory that cannot be tested (Table 1.6).

In addition to this vital flaw, I will repeat my assertion that education does not change the values held by students. We have overestimated the effect of public education. The gross association of the spread of education with the alteration of modern human attitudes has led us to suppose this. However this association has never been valid.

1.1.5 Demographic Transition Is Only a Tale and not a Theory

From its inception, demographic transition has been hypothetical. There are no countries that have actually experienced the course of demographic transition as described in the theory.

The British organization, Political and Economic Planning (PEP) developed a four phase model of demographic transition (see Fig. 1.2, p. 6) in 1960. This model only explains modern demographic change in simple and not theoretical terms. To begin with, there were no countries that accurately correspond to this model. The reason why it has been accepted is simply that it can be widely understood.

Now that we have grasped the fact that industrialization, urbanization, and education are not the causes of fertility decline, as previously thought, we should relinquish the theory of demographic transition and the development stage or evolution phase concept itself.

This old, demolished demographic theory can be replaced with reaction-diffusion theory, which I discuss later in this book. Here it should be noted that this alternative theory introduces a differential equation that allows for the falsifiability of the prediction.

1.1.5.1 Enhanced Nutritional Status and Not Demographic Transition Theory Explains the Decline of Mortality: McKeown's Thesis

Until now, I have exclusively examined fertility decline. However, the decline of mortality during the nineteenth century was not caused by the development of medicine and public health. This remarkable thesis was presented by Thomas McKeown [52] in 1962. McKeown published a series of controversial studies on the decline of mortality and population growth during the nineteenth and twentieth centuries in England and Wales [49–51].

Demographic transition theory postulates that the population increase during the late eighteenth and nineteenth centuries in England and Wales was caused by the decline of mortality induced by the development of medicine and public health. From the 1960s, this postulation has been questioned, for example, by Habakkuk [26] and Levine. Demographers and household economists have routinely ignored these questions to maintain the model of demographic transition.

McKeown presented the following propositions. First, the development of medical and public health measures had little to do with the decline in the death rate, and second, increasing food supplies led to enhanced nutritional status at the population level.

It was not until the discovery of antibiotics that medicine was able to effectively save lives. After World War II, for the first time, medicine was successful in saving lives. These facts make McKeown's ideas persuasive, further suggesting that modernization and industrialization during the nineteenth century were not the cause of the mortality decline.

It was not until 1900 that the infant mortality rate began to decline in England and Wales [1]. However fertility began to decline around 1870, or 1880 at the latest (from the index I_f by Coale, etc.). In England and Wales, too, fertility declined earlier than mortality decline. Demographic transition theory is thus also incongruous in the original context of the model and has been laid to rest. Moreover, the development stage theory is too simplistic to be considered realistic.

1.2 The Early Stage of Diffusion Hypothesis and Its Limitations

1.2.1 Carved Seals of Diffusion

Figures 1.4, 1.5, 1.6 and 1.7 depict maps of Europe with the shades of colors varying according to the level of I_g. I_g is an index of marital fertility calculated by Coale and his colleagues which measures marital fertility in comparison with the average marital fertility of Hutterites. A deeper shade of red expresses lower fertility, whereas a deeper shade of blue expresses higher fertility.

The diffusion of lower fertility rapidly spreads. However, geographical barriers prevented the spread of lower fertility. The Pyrenees mountain range historically constrained diffusion processes between France and Spain. However this barrier was circumvented and diffusion occurred in waves, penetrating Spain through a small gap alongside the Mediterranean Sea. We can precisely observe this circumventing wave.

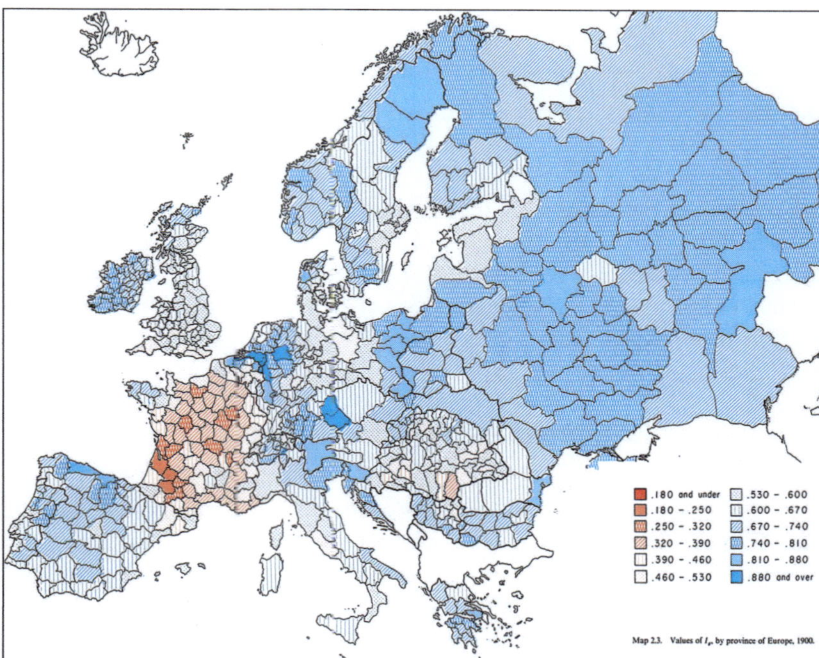

Fig. 1.5 Map 2.3. Values of I_g by province in Europe, 1900

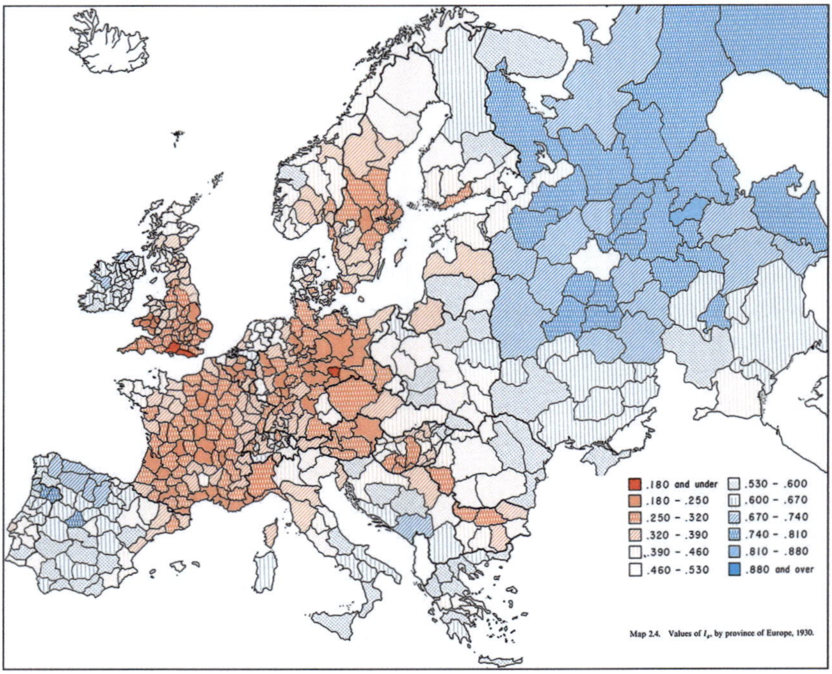

Fig. 1.6 Map 2.4. Values of I_g by province in Europe, 1930

Other mountain ranges, notably, the Alps and the Apennines also obstructed waves of lower fertility. These barriers constrained contact between people, and, therefore, blocked the diffusion of lowered fertility. The theory of fertility decline must explain these observed phenomena. The question is whether household economics can provide a reasonable explanation.

1.3 Household Economics—Not Even Wrong

From the 1980s, the diffusion hypothesis passed into oblivion in the shadow of household economics. Household economics appears to offer theoretical explanations for every demographic phenomenon. It reduces fertility decline to the subjective maximization of the expected utility of each set of parents.

Household economics posits that whether or not fertility decline occurs is contingent upon our subjective choices. Thus, demographic transition is a result of the simple aggregate of individual choices. This reasoning, while appearing to be valid, is in fact superficial and false, as illustrated by three decisive arguments described below.

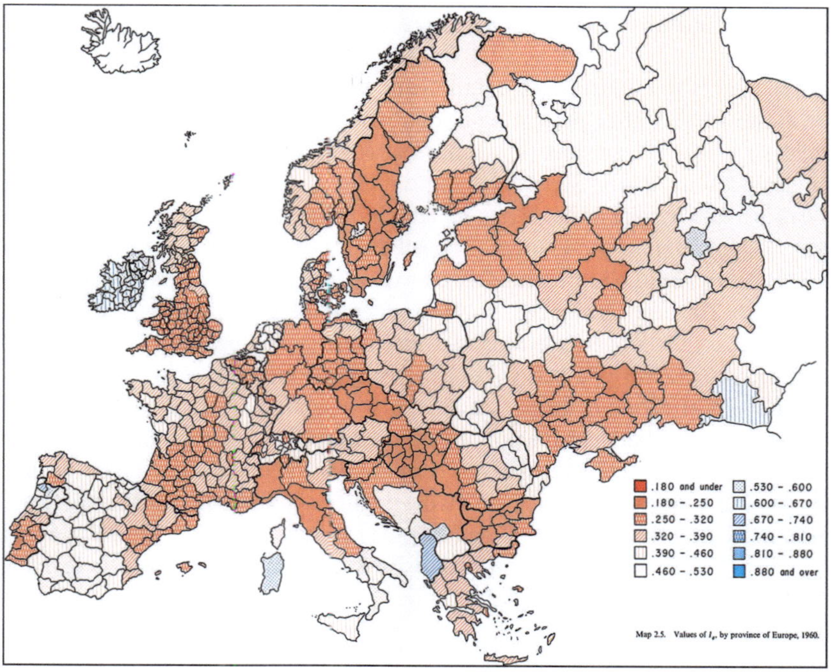

Fig. 1.7 Map 2.5. Values of I_g, by province in Europe, 1960. *Source* Fig. 1.4–1.7 from *The Decline of Fertility in Europe* [15]

1.3.1 Is a Society's Formation Entirely the Result of our Clear and Conscious Choices?

The first argument is that if the reasoning suggested by household economics is true, each set of parents would arbitrarily increase or reduce the number of children. This goes against our feeling of affection. Is a society completely the outcome of our clear and conscious choices? I think that such a conception lacks intellectual depth or knowledge, reducing social phenomena into subjective choices.

We become conscious of something entirely after an event. This post-event consciousness has a double meaning. One meaning concerns timing. We perceive an identified intention after we have initiated action. However, the vast realm of underconsciousness precedes action. Exploration of this unknown region is crucial for a discipline which genuinely asks questions. The argument that our conscious intentions decide our actions is a superficial one. We cannot assume the existence of an individual without neighbors. Nor can we assume the independent intention of an individual from his or her neighbors. Thus, we cannot construct society as a simple aggregate of individuals with intentions.

1.3.1.1 Alterations of Circumstances are Previous Given

There is another point that is more significant, scientific, and philosophical. We have to be aware and act after perceiving our circumstances. When we act appropriately in relation to our circumstances, we have a valid intention. This suggests that our circumstances are always superior to our consciousness. The alteration of our preferences is a false explanation. When no alteration of circumstances take place, there can be no alteration of preferences. The subjective apprehension of the intention to reduce the number of children is a flawed explanation and does not indicate a causal relationship. The aim of science is not to produce a likely explanation, but to discover unanticipated knowledge and to predict real changes in society based on accurate knowledge of causality. When we depend on preferences, we effectively lose the connection to effective causality. In line with evolutionary theory, the subjective intentions of living beings have no role in the causality of demographic phenomena.

The most important objective of any demographic theory is not to give credence to emotions, but rather to deduce the falsifiable prediction. The explanations provided by household economics have no computable possibilities, and their futility is evident. In other words, the explanations offered by household economics have no real utility and are misguided.

1.3.2 What Are the Causes of Alterations of Preferences?

My second argument is that while fertility decline is admittedly the result of alterations of parents' preferences in relation to children's qualities, in the final analysis, we must discover the underlying reasons for these alterations in preferences. Becker and his adherents eventually had to rely on appropriate changes in the "Background" in this regard.

They postulated that over time, background alterations such as industrialization, urbanization, the spread of education, and the spread of contraceptive methods or devices were the causes of fertility decline. However, such explanations are not only stereotyped, but also false, as we have previously shown.

In the previous section, we showed that no suitable and sufficient background alterations occurred during the period of demographic transition. Alterations of preferences are too superficial in general to explain reality, and are tautological. The hypothesis of household economics is negated both by observed data and by its illogical analysis. Truth-based theory demonstrates the unique property whereby it alone can explain a phenomenon. This is not the case with the explanation provided by the theory of revealed preferences. At most, this theory provides a veneer of commonplace knowledge.

By contrast, diffusion theory entails a strong element of surprise. It compels a re-examination of human behavior. The most essential causal element is the number of children of the neighbors of each set of parents and not the background. Diffusion theory enables us to abandon the concept of a "modern" independent person who accurately assesses background conditions.

1.3.3 The Lack of Falsifiability

My third argument is closely associated with the above argument. First, though, we should ask whether the alteration of preferences hypothesis has ever been verified. Preferences cannot be measured and examined, which are required for their verification. They are intangible and used to explain human consciousness. Preferences always only apply to explanations and do not contribute to predictions. There is no evidence of the alteration of preferences in the process of demographic transition. Scientific theories must be falsifiable. Accordingly, household economics does not provide a scientific theory, because it only offers justifications and cannot contribute falsifiable predictions.

The explanation that an alteration of preferences results in a reduction in the number of children is a tautology. Imagining an action always precedes a subjective intention.

There is no decisive way of testing the validity of the alteration of preferences hypothesis. It is, therefore, surprising that this weak logic has acquired authority. It appeals to subjectivity for its plausibility. However, science cannot be built on human subjectivity. The effect of our thinking is no evidence at all.

1.3.4 Not Even Wrong

Becker did not apply mathematical induction to prove inequalities. Consequently, he explained a marriage outcome as follows.

> If Z_{m0} and Z_{0f} represent the maximum outputs of single M and F, and m_{mf} and f_{mf} their incomes when married, a necessary condition for M and F to marry is that
>
> $$m_{mf} \geq Z_{m0} \qquad (8)$$
> $$f_{mf} \geq Z_{0f}.$$
>
> If $m_{mf} + f_{mf}$, the total income produced by the marriage, is identified with the output of the marriage, a necessary condition for marriage is the that
>
> $$m_{mf} + f_{mf} \equiv Z_{mf} \geq Z_{m0} + Z_{0f}. \qquad (9)$$
>
> Since most men and women over age 20 are married in all societies, equation (9) must generally hold because of fundamental reasons that are not unique to time or place. I have a useful framework for discovering these reasons.
>
> G.S. Becker [2], pp. 209–210.

Becker's explanation is a typical tautology. He should have explained how marriages occur. The object to be explained is phenomenon A which is that most men and women over the age of 20 are married in all societies. He then introduced equation (9) (Proposition B) as a causal factor for occurrences of marriage. He thus used the generality of phenomenon A to prove the validity of Proposition B. The universality of marriage, which is the phenomenon to be explained, is not in fact explained at all. When Becker introduced the necessary conditions, he simply assumed the universality of occurrences of marriage. This unexamined introduction of the necessary condition is entirely doubtful. It should be possible to prove whether the necessary condition (8), which is a hypothesis, is true or false. We should be able to deduce the validity of equation (9) with another Proposition C, which is widely accepted.

Let me note in passing that Becker's necessary condition (9) has historically been disproved because some societies have men and women over the age of 20 who are not married. I find it difficult to believe that this weakly argued and tautological argument has endured for decades.

Some of his other explanations are also inaccurate.

> If each person is a utility maximizer and choose the mate who maximize his utility, the optimal sorting must have the property that persons not married to each other could not marry without making at least one of them worse off. In game theoritic language, the optimal sorting is in the core, since no(monogamous) coalition outside the core could make either of its member better off without making the other worth off.
>
> G.S. Becker [3], p. 68.

The core is solely proved by its existence within game theory. However, it is not always achieved in actual games. Once a coalition has been formed, nobody leaves the core. However, whether or not we can accomplish the core cannot be proved. In fact the probability of accomplishing the core is negligible. In addition to this insurmountable problem, the core is not unique. If we admit to an indifferent order, there may be thousands of cores within a large marriage market. Thus, in general, game theory is unable to produce predictions.

Within the core, why does divorce occur? The response of household economists is that there is incomplete information available. However, the completeness, accuracy, and validity of information are assumed within ordinal game theory. Household economists thus offer an excuse instead of a prediction. They simply insist that real marriage is the core without providing any empirical grounds for this. I, therefore, argue that the hypothesis proposed by household economists is not even wrong. This is because their insistence is faith-based and is not even a hypothesis.

Household economics is a pseudo-science, because its underlying logic is weak and the proofs offered are entirely inaccurate.

1.3.4.1 The Quantity and Quality of Children is not Falsifiable

Becker insisted that the decline in the number of the children of each set of parents resulted from a shift in preference from quantity to quality. This argument too is tautological.

> The analysis is then extended to consider the interaction between quantity and quality of children, probably the major contribution of the economic analysis of fertility. This interaction

> explains why the quantity of children often changes rapidly over time even though there are no close substitutes for children and the income elasticity is not large.
>
> G.S. Becker [3], p. 93.

If Becker's argument was not tautological, he would have been able to predict how an interaction that occurred between quantity and quality would influence the decline in the number of children of each set of parents. It is impossible for household economists to distribute this prediction, because they have no concrete and calculable equations for this problem. They only have suggestive and plausible indifferent curves.

A more complicated and pedantic expression of the concept of interaction between the quantity and quality of children is the subjective alteration of motivation which is widely assumed. This "stopgap" concept is of no use in revolutionary discovery. Becker's analysis was, at the most, ordinary knowledge.

What causes an alteration of the interaction between the quantity and quality of children? Becker did not discuss alterations of socioeconomic conditions. Background alterations were assumed. However, there are no decisive relations between fertility decline and background. They believe somehow so it seems to go. Such shallow thinking cannot arrive at the truth.

The concept of interaction between the quantity and quality of children cannot produce a falsifiable prediction. Yet, Becker wrote that this concept had made a major contribution to the economic analysis of fertility. However, the genuine value of the economic analysis of fertility can be easily discerned, the veneer of academic knowledge.

1.3.4.2 Decisive Evidence is Logically Impossible

Some may consider my criticism to be extraordinarily exaggerated. There are many prudent scholars and academics who consider household economics to be reasonable. However, a majority does not equal the truth.

Such scholars argue that the intention to act may be subjective. In these cases, we may easily succumb to the illusion of trying to explain this intention causally. The causal agency of intentions put forward is that these are automatic patterns of our recognition. We cannot observe the intentions of others without the action. That is to say, the action itself occurs earlier than the intention for an observer. We are able to scientifically and empirically postulate just the action itself, but this is categorically impossible for the intention. An intention is mere conjecture, which is a common attribute of people. However, our intentions are not scientific objects.

Because of our similarities as individuals, our conjectures are almost identical. However, there is no evidence that our conjectures regarding our intentions are correct, and that they truly preexist actions.[1] However, this is still not proof of the

[1] See B. Libet [47]. Libet provided empirical evidence that our brains start to act before we acquire consciousness.

existence of subjective intentions. Scientific theory must be built on an empirical and not a reflective base. The conception of revealed preferences is not adequate for constructing a scientific theory. Such a theory must be based on observable phenomena.

The likelihood of our sensitivity is by no means decisive evidence. We must confine the meaning of evidence for a theory to that whereby it enables a calculable prediction to be deduced and tested with observed data. Household economics has not provided us with any calculable predictions.

Our subjective intentions, or preferences, are altered depending on the socioeconomic background. We have no ability to predict how the socioeconomic background will be altered. Consequently, when we presume background dependence of fertility, it is a hopeless task to attempt to predict future fertility.

When our subjective intentions and preferences are posited as ultimate causes, it is impossible for us to predict them. In principle, we prefer arbitrariness.

Our subjective intentions and preferences are, therefore, mere consequences of our actions. We are fortunate that our actions are solely dependent on our actions with respect to fertility decline as described in chapter two.

1.4 Evidence of Background Independence

We can find ample evidence that fertility declined independently from its background context. I have already shown that education did not affect fertility decline in Japan. I will now introduce other evidences in the context of Japan, and which effectively demonstrate the features of diffusion.

1.4.1 Japan

In Japan, fertility declined[2] synchronously in Tokyo and Osaka from the beginning of the twentieth century (see Fig. 1.8 and Table 1.7). It should be noted that Tokyo is situated at a distance of around 400 km from Osaka (see Fig. 1.9).

In contrast to this simultaneity with regard to the decline in the number of children per couple in Osaka and Tokyo, the backgrounds of these two cities differ significantly. Osaka's infant death rate was much higher than that of Tokyo (see Table 1.8). Despite evidencing the highest infant death rate in Japan, Osaka was the the first Japanese prefecture where fertility decline was evident.

More astonishingly, the fertility decline in Osaka occurred in spite of the fact that the infant death rate was still increasing in 1920 (this corresponds to the 1890 cohort). In spite of the evident risk of having fewer children than before, couples reduced the number of their children. An individual does not think about the future as an outcome of his or her own decisions. Thus, the hypothesis of demographic

[2]The number of children per couple declined from around 1900 to 1960.

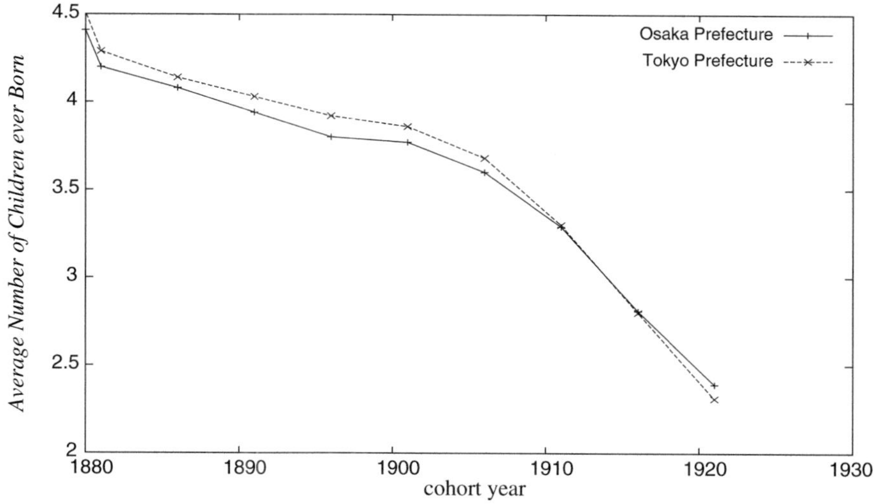

Fig. 1.8 Fertility decline in Tokyo and Osaka

Table 1.7 Fertility decline in Tokyo and Osaka (numeric data)

Cohort	Osaka total	Osaka in the densely-inhabited district	Osaka Kita-ku	Tokyo total	Tokyo in the densely-inhabited district	Chiyoda-ku
Before 1880	4.41	4.39	4.01	4.51	4.42	3.84
1881–1885	4.20	4.11	3.87	4.29	4.21	3.94
1886–1890	4.08	3.96	3.84	4.14	4.03	3.72
1891–1895	3.94	3.84	3.44	4.03	3.92	3.48
1896–1900	3.80	3.69	3.29	3.92	3.79	3.50
1901–1905	3.77	3.49	3.30	3.86	3.75	3.19
1906–1910	3.60	3.49	3.15	3.68	3.58	3.18
1911–1915	3.29	3.18	2.79	3.30	3.22	2.95
1916–1920	2.81	2.74	2.50	2.80	2.74	2.67
1921–1925	2.39	2.34	2.15	2.31	2.27	2.16

**Source* Population Census of Japan 1960, 1970

transition theory that each set of parents reduces the number of their children as a reaction to a decline in the death rate is an overestimation and illusion. I suggest that the alteration of mortality did not affect the decline of fertility in Japan (Table 1.9).

Other background differences between Tokyo and Osaka did not affect fertility decline. Table 1.10 shows that the educational level of females in Tokyo was much higher than that of females in Osaka. Traditional demographic transition theory suggests that education attainment encourages fertility decline. This implies that the decline of fertility in Tokyo should have preceded that in Osaka. However, fertility decline occurred simultaneously in these cities. Moreover, around 1900, Tokyo was an eastern hub and Japan's capital, and was developing at a faster pace than Osaka.

Fig. 1.9 A map of Japan

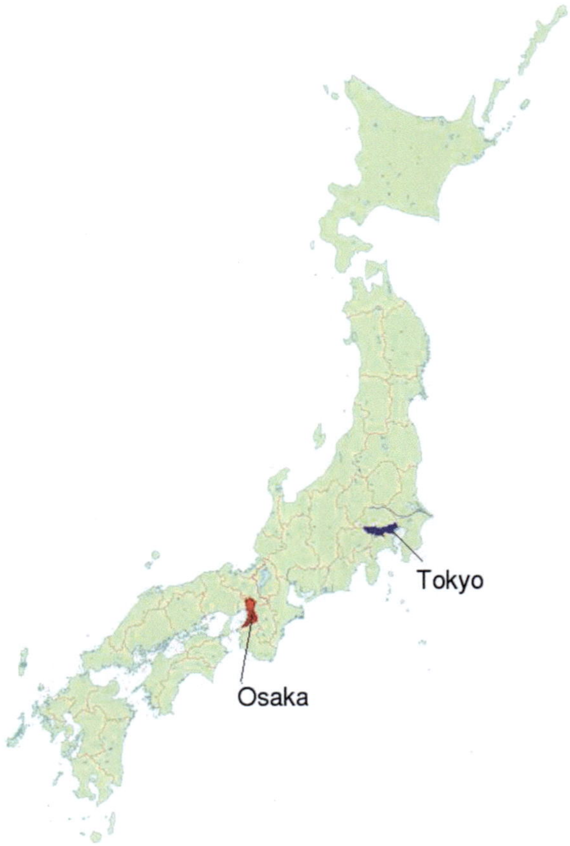

The rate of participation of women in the labor force, by industry, differed significantly in Tokyo and Osaka (see Table 1.9). Tokyo was much more modernized than Osaka. However, fertility in the two cities declined at almost the same tempo.[3] A valid theory of fertility decline must be able to describe this synchronicity independently from its background.

These facts suggest that individuals do not react to background socioeconomic alterations. They respond solely to the number of children evident among other sets of parents. The simultaneity observed in Tokyo and Osaka can be reasonably explained by this process of individuals responding to others.

It is notable that there are multiple (at least two) origins of diffusion in Japan.

---

[3]Some may argue that this simultaneity contradicts the diffusion hypothesis. It is impossible for diffusion to occur instantly so that a phenomenon occurs simultaneously in two places located at a distance of 400 km from each other. At the end of the nineteenth century, however, the diffusion process had evolved to a new phase, enabling fertility decline to diffuse to remote points by means of advances in transportation.

Table 1.8 Infant death rate from 1920 to 1929 in Tokyo and Osaka

	Tokyo	Osaka
1920	167.6	223.8
1921	163.5	229.8
1922	158.6	236.7
1923	175.6	218.6
1924	152.3	185.9
1925	145.3	160.5
1926	129.2	155.0
1927	150.9	160.7
1928	132.6	168.8
1929	123.9	147.8

Note Calculations derived from *Kokusei chosa igo Nihon jinko tokei shusei* [45]

Table 1.9 Percentages of employees by industries in Tokyo and Osaka

Research year	Percentage of female employees in all industries				
	Agriculture	Manufacturing	Service	Financial and insurance	Official
Tokyo					
1920	12.77	27.68	39.85	0.04	0.62
1930	8.29	17.06	44.45	0.94	1.17
1950	8.77	23.63	27.62	3.62	3.94
Research year	Percentage of female employees in all industries				
	Agriculture	Manufacturing	Service	Financial and insurance	Official
Osaka					
1920	14.01	39.25	27.45	0.41	0.27
1930	12.32	24.50	28.63	0.77	0.44
1950	12.04	33.84	20.00	2.67	2.45

Source Sangyo betu Shugyou sha no jikeiretu hikaku, Sourihu Toukei Kyouku [62]

Table 1.10 Female educational levels in Tokyo and Osaka in 1950 (aged 25 plus and not in school)

Percent	0 year	1–6	7–12	13 or more	Unknown
Tokyo	4.0	32.9	58.5	4.6	0.1
Osaka	7.1	39.4	51.0	2.5	0.0

**Source Teikoku Tokei Nenkan* Population Census of Japan 1950

1.4.2 Normal Distribution in Hokaido

Diffusion proceeds as normal distribution with an increase in variance. Fick's law and Fourier's law both come down to the normal distribution, mathematically. The mathematical solution of the diffusion model by Fick's law and Fourier's law is the normal distribution.

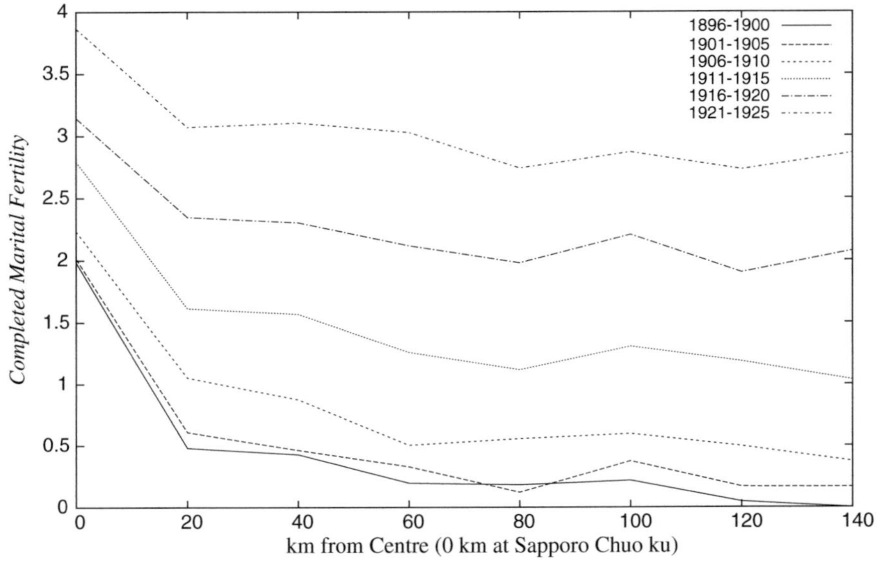

Fig. 1.10 Longitudinal changes of the index in Hokkaido

I found a semi-normal distribution based on the transformation equation shown below in Hokkaido, Japan.

$$6.474 - \text{Average number of children in each town and village} \tag{1.1}$$

6.474 is the max of the average number of children in Hokkaido.

I plotted a graph from the point of origin (Saporo) to the towns and villages located along concentric circles (see Fig. 1.10). We can see that fertility decline in Hokkaido showed a normal distribution with an increase in variance. This is clearly evidence of the diffusion of fertility decline.

1.5 The Rise of Neo-Diffusionism

The rise of neo-diffusionism was evident by the end of the twentieth century. M.R. Montgomery and J.B. Casterline wrote an article entitled, "The diffusion of fertility control in Taiwan: Evidence from pooled cross-section time-series models" [54]. This article explained fertility decline in Taiwan primarily from the perspective of the diffusion of fertility control methods. They included maps (Fig. 1.11), which demonstrate the diffusion process. When observing fertility decline (mainly in terms of numbers of children) in developing countries, we must map the diffusion process. Such maps were earlier constructed by the Princeton European Fertility Project on

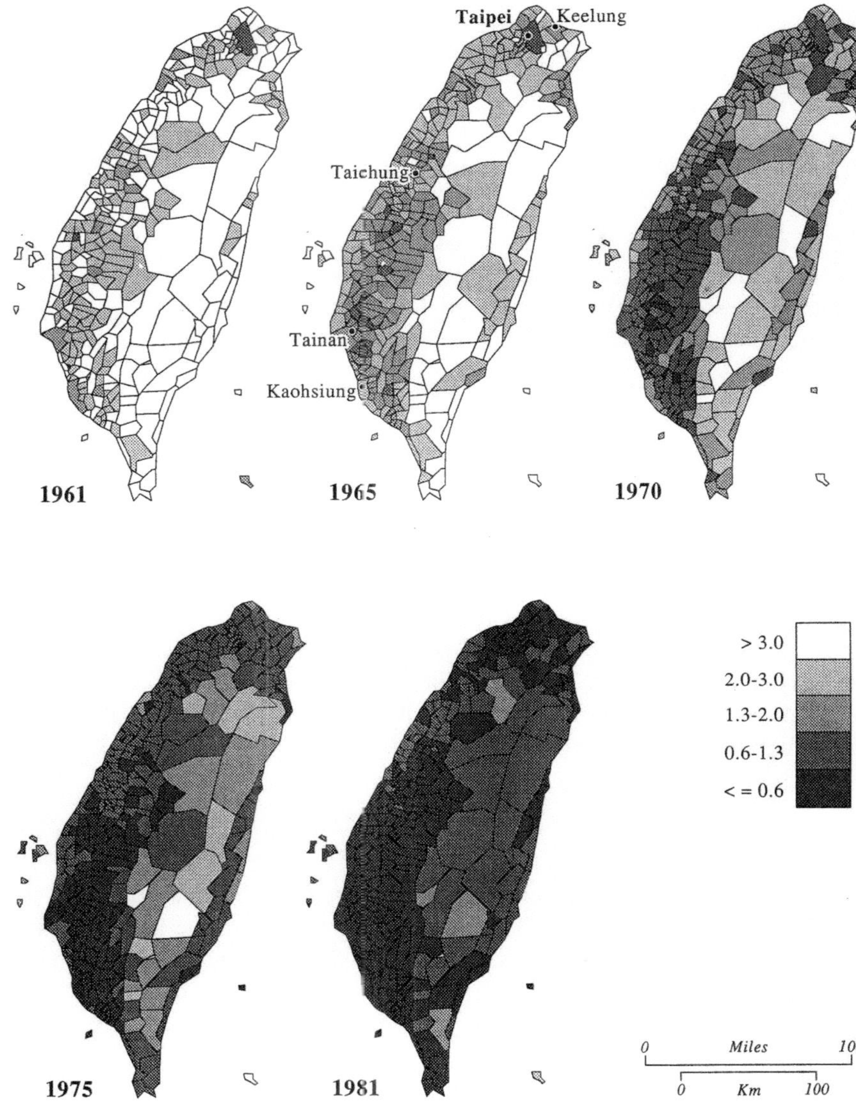

Fig. 1.11 Fertility decline in Taiwan

which the diffusion process was superimposed. This raises the question of how and why this clear evidence has been ignored for several decades.

The phenomenon of diffusion cannot be denied. For this, the credit goes to Montgomery and Casterline. However I do not agree with their argument regarding the mechanism of diffusion. Montgomery and Casterline attributed diffusion to the "learning of contraceptive methods" [55]. While the explanation that contraceptive methods diffused through learning is indeed plausible, in terms of scientific reasoning, the plausibility of the explanation may be liable to error.

1.5.1 Mathematical Model of Neo-Diffusionism

The logistic model proposed by the neo-diffusionists does not explicitly contain a diffusion mechanism. A diffusion hypothesis must be formulated based on concrete diffusion processes. This implies that the diffusion model of low fertility has to incorporate Fick's law of diffusion. In the mathematical formulation, the diffusion term $D\dfrac{\partial^2 C}{\partial x^2}$ must be included in the equation.

1.5.2 The Model of Rosero-Bixby and Casterline

At the end of the twentieth century, J.B. Casterline and his colleagues presented a micro dynamic model and statistical analysis of diffusion.

Rosero-Bixby and Casterline [59] revived the diffusion hypothesis by applying a mathematical model that the older diffusionists lacked. Their model combined the model proposed by J.S. Coleman for the spread of innovation with the logistic model.

Their differential equation is shown below.

$$\frac{dY_t}{dt} = a(L - Y_t) + hY_t(L - Y_t) \tag{1.2}$$

Y_t expresses the ratio of the population that have accepted the innovation. L is the limit of Y. The ratio of the population that have not accepted the innovation is a proportional determinative of the development Y with coefficient a. The first nomial is Coleman's spread of innovation. Rosero-Bixby and Casterline regarded the first nomial as an effect of the enlightenment campaign by means of messages transmitted through the mass media.

The second nomial is the logistic model, while h is a coefficient that determines the speed of spread. In contrast to the monotonous effect of the first nomial, the effect of this logistic nomial Y results in an inflection point.

1.5.2.1 The Coleman Nomial is Unnecessary

This mixed model of diffusion is easy to understand and is plausible. However, it does not provide an answer to the question of how the number of children of each set of parents is decided. Does an awareness campaign conducted through the mass media have any effects? I predict that messages conveyed through the mass media do not influence the process of fertility decline. At the level of the nation state, we are only able to fit the logistic curve to the observed data. The inclusion of Coleman's nomial is, therefore, quite unnecessary.

Rosero-Bixby and Casterline arrived at their difference equation (1.3) by applying the Euler method to their differential equation (1.2).[4]

$$Y_t = aL + (1 - a + hL)Y_{t-1} - hY_{t-1}{}^2 \tag{1.3}$$

Rosero-Bixby and Casterline interpreted the logistic nomial as an expression of contagious diffusion. However, we should reflect on what contagion is within the process of fertility decline. They did not think through the process of contagious diffusion by considering relevant questions such as where this occurs.

This weakness of their model can be attributed to their difference equation. Below, I expand the brackets of Eq. (1.3) and incorporate Y_{t-1} within it.

$$Y_t = aL + (1 - a + hL - hY_{t-1})Y_{t-1}$$

Let me now rearrange the bracketed portion of the equation, paying attention to h.

$$Y_t = aL + h(L + \frac{1-a}{h} - Y_{t-1})Y_{t-1} \tag{1.4}$$

We cannot reasonably interpret this difference equation. The meanings of the coefficients are unclear. The true mathematical expression of objects does not entail the loss of their meaning.

1.5.3 The Background-Dependent Simultaneous Differential Equation Model

Rosero-Bixby and Casterline enhanced their model to apply it to a heterogeneous population that was divided into two strata with three states: (N (natural fertility), L (latent demand) and C (birth control).

They explained this as follows.

> Demand factors(shaped by structural and cultural conditions) drive the flow between state N and L; supply factors(shaped in part by programme interventions) drive the flow between L and C.
>
> Rosero-Bixby and Casterline, Modeling Diffusion Effects in Fertility Transition [59], p. 165

However, this enhancement is entirely metaphorical. There is no need to divide a population into two strata; nor into three states. Their model is eclectic and too complex to yield any falsifiable predictions.

---

[4]Coefficients *a and h* are altered to other values.

Differential fertility across social strata is plausible. However no significant differences in fertility between social strata are currently evident in Japan. In western European countries, there is also no difference across social strata. The slight difference is reduced to the difference in the continuous length of marriages.

In the process of fertility decline in Europe, class differentiated fertility is not so important.

> For example, evidence on class differentials from England shows a widening of differences during the early decades of the transition, but significant falls occurring in almost all social classes about the same. Similarly, to quote Watkins once more, evidence from other countries indicates that, although fertility decline may be most dramatic in urban, industrial, educated populations, 'The effect of modernization need not be confined to those individuals who adopt new occupations, who move to the city, who learn to read.' Transition theories usually predict that some groups will find birth control advantageous and others disadvantageous on economic grounds. However, as Watkins notes, the European evidence suggests that, whatever the economics, 'even those who could be expected to find continued childbearing advantageous or family limitation unacceptable adopted family limitation rather quickly after the leaders'.
>
> J. Cleland and C. Wilson [8], p. 24.

Rosero-Bixby and Casterline thought that diffusion was caused by demand factors (shaped by structural and cultural conditions) related to the "background" context of the diffusion process. They posited that whether or not diffusion occurred depended on human subjective motivations that were shaped by structural and cultural conditions. This conventional and commonplace solution in fact solved nothing as it lacked a law-like nature. Moreover, their simultaneous differential equations were no more than demonstrations.

They assumed that learning was the main factor in the transition from L to C. They further supposed that the alteration of demand caused by the background was mediated by learning about contraception.

1.5.3.1 Learning is not the Cause of Diffusion

There is critical counterevidence against the explanation offered by Rosero-Bixby and Casterline. At the onset of fertility decline in Europe around the end of the eighteenth century, there were no effective contraceptive methods available. Moreover, fertility decline had already begun in the southwest of France. This implies that the number of children per set of parents declined without the use of any effective contraceptive methods. Effective contraceptive methods were therefore not a necessary condition for fertility decline.

It is not necessary to assume a transition from state L to state C.

As Malthus asserted, fertility is controlled by practicing continence. When each set of parents controls their fertility, there is no need for learning. H.P. Kohler maintained that parents located within social networks learn about the use of contraception [40]. His argument, while plausible, is also untenable.

A decline in fertility occurred in Hungary before 1890 (see Table 1.1). Almost all Hungarians had no access to contraceptive utilities at that time, because Hungary remained an agricultural country that was dependent on human power. There was also no necessity for them to control their fertility as a prerequisite for birth control.

> Although the fertility decline began in England only after considerable urbanization and industrialization had taken place, it occurred at about the same time in Hungary, which was at a substantially lower level of development as measured by conventional socioeconomic indexes.
>
> J. Knodel and Etienne van de Walle [36], pp. 223–224

The primary issue here is that Rosero-Bixby and Casterline did not clearly define what is learned by parents. The objectives of learning can only be imagined by readers based on the implicit background.

We have already seen that no consistent cross-sectional or cross-chronological modifications of background occurred in the process of fertility decline. In other words, the neo-diffusionists cannot clarify "what is learned."

They seem to be unable to forsake the well-worn obsession that we adapt to background alterations by means of learning.

1.6 The True Impact of Diffusion Hypothesis: Background Independence

Rosero-Bixby and Casterline appear to have forgotten what was earlier noted by the older-diffusionists, namely, that there were no reasonable and uniform demands in the process of diffusion.

> In the European experience, the connection between socio-economic structural change and fertility decline also was rather loose. Within remarkably short span of time, fertility transition occurred in both economically more advanced and less advanced countries.
>
> J. Knodel [37], p. 246

A diffusion model that is background-dependent is compromised, although this error on the part of Rosero-Bixby and Casterline was not consciously made. They just did not understand the profound impact of diffusion, and implicitly assumed that couples were consciously aware of their motivations to control their fertility. This assumption, however, is simplistic. The true impact of diffusion is that the diffusion process itself generates demand factors (motivations) so that we can omit them. I refer to this distinctive quality of diffusion as "background independence."

If diffusion depends on demand factors (shaped by structural and cultural conditions), we cannot predict the diffusion process until we can understand how structural and cultural conditions generate and alter these factors. It is apparent that we cannot conceive how structural and cultural conditions generate and alter these factors.

Building a genuine social science in this background dependence manner is a desperate measure. We must renounce the classical idea that demand factors are dependent on socioeconomic background.

Is subjective demand a prerequisite for birth control? Why is this postulated within a social science without any definite proof of its existence? It is, after all, only a subjective conception.

The true significance of the diffusion process is its automatic development. The demand for birth control is consciously or unconsciously manifested when couples become aware that their neighbors are having fewer children. Our desire comes about only when we compare ourselves with our neighbors. Preferences are revealed only after we recognize others' conditions. The concept of revealed preference regarding the number of children in household economics is, therefore, false and does not make sense. This is because we cannot have preferences in the absence of knowledge regarding the number of children of our neighbors.

When we incorporate the number of neighboring children into our model of diffusion, we automatically solve the demand problem.

What is more important for the diffusion model is to concretely, deliberately, and spatially draw out the real diffusion process in relation to the number of children that couples have. For this purpose, it is necessary to construct a geographical diffusion model because the observed phenomena are geographical in nature. Without considering this factor, the diffusion model is only an esquisse.

The commonplace nature of the model proposed by Rosero-Bixby and Casterline is the result of its omission of "background independence," which is the true essence of diffusion.

Moreover, they did not construct a mathematical model of diffusion. Their pooled cross-section time-series models amount to no more than regression models. However, a statistical regression model cannot be used to deduce a falsifiable prediction. Neo-diffusionists were unable to construct a mathematical diffusion model, and thus postulated plausible background modifications for diffusion by means of parents learning and adapting to them.

1.6.1 A Preoccupation Which Governs Us

We have been obsessed by the preoccupation that socioeconomic conditions determine the number of children selected by each set of parents, subjectively and independently from other sets of parents. This preoccupation is merely ideological and has not been empirically proven.

Is it true that our behavior follows our conscious cogitation? Do we conduct ourselves after experiencing background alterations?

The diffusion hypothesis is the most probable explanation for these phenomena that occur without any preoccupation. It should be considered as a scientific theory, because it is described by an equation and can produce falsifiable predictions.

When we admit the assumption that a set of parents is influenced by neighboring sets of parents, we are able to deduce falsifiable predictions from a well formulated equation.

In contrast to the falsifiability of the diffusion hypothesis, the explanation offered by household economics is simply an explanation that cannot be verified, because it cannot produce verifiable predictions. Household economics is not a science. It is only an explanation and is, therefore, not even wrong.

1.7 What Diffusion Theory Should Propose

The validity of diffusion theory must be demonstrated by finding evidence that can only be explained by the diffusion process. By evidence, I mean predictions that are deduced from a mathematical diffusion model of fertility decline and which is positively tested through empirical procedure. Plausible eclecticism does not lead to the Promised Land.

A valid diffusion theory must deduce falsifiable predictions independently from the background context. The fertility decline in Europe and Japan occurred independently from the background. What claims to be scientific theory must be expressible by an equation that involves falsifiable predictions.

Here, I introduce the features that diffusion theory should possess. The first *irreversibility* has been pointed out by the early diffusionists. In the upsurge of household economics, the rational choice crusaders eliminated these features almost unconsciously. Cleland and Wilson mentioned the second feature of *stability and smoothing* as something to be resisted against them.

1.7.1 Irreversibility

Fertility decline is an irreversible process. The early diffusionists clearly described this feature as follows.

> Increases in the practice of family limitation and the decline of marital fertility were largely coincident and, once under way, were largely irreversible and gained momentum.
>
> J. Knodel and E. van de Walle, *op. cit.*, p. 232

Thus, a valid theory of fertility decline must include this feature of irreversibility.

1.7.2 Stability and Smoothing

Cleland and Wilson noted the following important features of diffusion. When fertility decline has advanced, there is no divergence in the preferred numbers of children between different cohorts.

> A cross-national analysis of WFS[5] data by Lighbourne and MacDonald gives a similar impression. When the number of living children was controlled, they found no evidence of divergence in preferred numbers of children in different cohorts of women. They conclude that either historical shifts in family size norms or desires have affected all generations equally (which is possible , but seems unlikely) or that desires have remained stable.
>
> J. Cleland and C. Wilson [8], pp. 25–26.

I will elaborate on this feature. There is no divergence either by profession or by income strata. According to modern statistical data, average numbers of children in western European countries are very similar and stable. A valid theory of fertility decline must, therefore, also incorporate stability and the smoothing effect.

[5]World Fertility Survey.

Chapter 2
Reaction-Diffusion of the Number of Children

Abstract When we admit the background independence of fertility decline and aspects of diffusion, we can construct a reaction-diffusion model to describe fertility decline as a stochastic process independent of its background. Once we postulate a reaction-diffusion process for this phenomenon, we can estimate the velocity of a progressive wave of diffusion. By means of the estimated velocity, we can estimate where a singularity of fertility decline was and when it appeared. The singularity existed in a French district *Aquitaine* basin. From *Lot-et-Garonne* in *Aquitaine* the reaction-diffusion of fertility decline began to diffuse to all Europe maintaining independence of socio-economic conditions.

Keywords Fertility decline · Reaction-diffusion · Singularity · Progressive wave · Stochastic limit · Aquitaine · Lot-et-Garonne

It is the most suitable solution for the predictions falsifiable to make Reaction-Diffusion System as background independent. It is essential and crucial to know the stochastic causality of the spatial number of children for the theory of fertility decline. Motivations of birth control are trifling even though they seems primal for our subjectivity.

2.1 What Is the Reaction-Diffusion System?

I introduce the “reaction-diffusion system” briefly. Reaction-diffusion systems are used to explain the development of various patterns or structures in space such as black hole, organs of organic body, and geographic undulations of fertility. A.M. Turing [65] insisted that the differential equation such as Eq. (2.1) or Eq. (2.7) consists of diffusion term and nonlinear development term describes various patterns of processes by means of their interactions.

$$\frac{\partial f(x,t)}{\partial t} = \frac{\partial^2 f(x,t)}{\partial x^2} + g(f(x,t)) \tag{2.1}$$

S. Ike, *Fertility Decline and Background Independence*,
Population Studies of Japan, DOI 10.1007/978-4-431-55151-5_2

The first term is a normal diffusion term. x is a parameter of space. t is a time. In reaction-diffusion system, "reaction" correspond to nonlinear development term $g(f(x,t))$. Reaction is rather an acceleration effect to a process. Reaction-diffusion system describes the development of f in a space by time.

Let us compare reaction-diffusion equation to McKendrick-von-Foerster equation well-known in Demography.

$$\frac{\partial p(t,a)}{\partial t} + \frac{\partial p(t,a)}{\partial a} = -\mu(a)p(t,a) \tag{2.2}$$

McKendrick equation describes the dynamics of the age structure $p(t,a)$ by mortality by age $\mu(a)$ and itself. In contrast with this, reaction-diffusion system pays no attention to the age structure of a given population. Containing a space parameter x in second order in the reaction-diffusion equation, the density-gradient plays a main role. Reaction-diffusion equation of the number of children describes solely how low fertility spreads and forms some pattern in a given space. In the first place R.A. Fisher [25] proposed RDE (Reaction–Diffusion Equation) in 1937 to describe how the advantageous genes spread in the space. Namely RDE congenitally equipes the ability to describe spacial fertility decline.

2.2 Reaction-Diffusion of the Number of Children

The first proposition that I introduce is that parents decide stochastically the number of children they will have under the influence of parents in their neighbourhood.

Proposition 2.1 NDISD (Neighbourhood Dependent Isotropic Stochastic Decision) *The number of children of each set of parents is isotropically and stochastically dependent on neighbouring numbers of children.*

We have good reason to suppose that the number of children is a stochastic variable. The indirect empirical evidence is that the completed marital fertility is almost proportional to the age when she married. L. Henry [28] observed this phenomena. When we assume that conceptions occur randomly, this proportionality is easily derived from this assumption.[1] So parents' decisions have fluctuations and a variance caused by them. If we calculate the number of children of parents under constant socio-economic conditions, we must observe fluctuations and a variance caused by them.

[1] Let p be a probability of a conception at a moment. $\int_0^t pdt$ is the number of children for t time. $\int_0^t pdt \equiv p(t+C)$.

As for the neighbourhood dependency, it is difficult to show empirical evidences here. When we admit this proposition, we can describe how high fertility changes to lower fertility, namely how relative lower fertility in a spot diffuses to other more fertile areas. After all, the validity of the neighbourhood dependency should be evaluated by this article itself. The discovery of a singularity of fertility decline can never be done without this assumption.

No one can deny that we receive influences form neighbouring others. I think NDISD is much more reliable than the doubtful revealed preference hypothesis.

2.2.1 Diffusion of Low Fertility

Consider parents distributed in one dimensional space (a linear habitat) divided into segments. Each segment has a value c which represents a level of fertility of parents resident in its segment. Normally we think c is a mean of the number of children of all sets of parents in a segment.

In the latter parts of this article, I consider higher dimensional spaces, so each segment will be rectangle in two or three dimensional space.

See Fig. 2.1. Let us conduct a "thought experiment" about what interaction takes place between a high fertility segment $c(x_0)$ and a neighbouring low fertility segment $c(x_{-1})$ in time. A segment $c(x_0)$ whose fertility is higher and a segment $c(x_{-1})$ whose fertility is lower affect each other, so that high fertility of $c(x_0)$ shifts to lower than before and low fertility of $c(x_{-1})$ shifts to higher. These alterations occur because parents in each segment stochastically affect each other.

Let us think, in Fig. 2.1, precisely and iteratively by time t_k about segments $c(x_{i-2}, t_0)$, $c(x_{i-1}, t_0)$ whose fertility is lower and about segments $c(x_{i+0}, t_0)$, $c(x_{i+1}, t_0)$ whose fertility is higher at time $t = 0$.

At $t = 1, c(x_{i-1}, t_1)$ rises, $c(x_{i+0}, t_1)$ descends. Next at $t = 2, c(x_{i-1}, t_2)$ rises and $c(x_{i+0}, t_2)$ descends exceedingly, along with these $c(x_{i-2}, t_2)$ rises and $c(x_{i+1}, t_2)$ descends a little. Between time t_0 to t_2 (for two unit of time), low fertility progressed from x_{i-2} to x_{i+1}. Thus low fertility have progressed three segments. These processes will be continued until there are no undulations to be smoothed.

In this simple "thought experiment", we can recognise three characteristics of historical fertility decline that is : *irreversibility, stability, and smoothing*. In addition

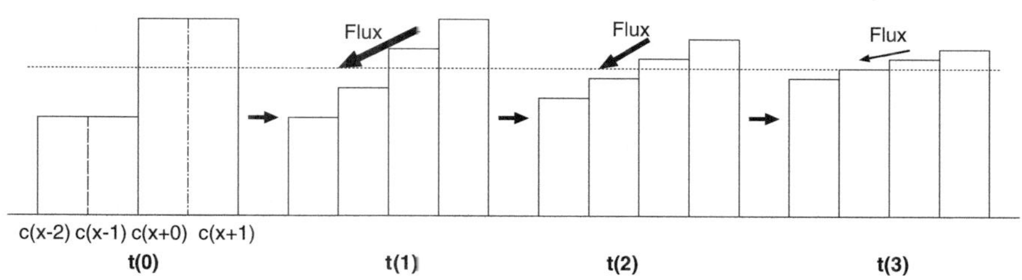

Fig. 2.1 When high fertility group contact to low fertility group

to them, we can see how a "progressive wave" moves. That is to say stochastic fluctuations of the number of children of parents convey lower fertility.

2.2.1.1 Not Imitation nor a Meme

Someone may consider this conveyance of lower fertility by stochastic fluctuations as "Imitation". This understanding is not precise. In the process of fertility decline, rarely some parents imitate the number of neighbouring parents consciously. However an overwhelmingly majority of parents did not have such affection. They consciously and originally decide their number of children taking into account neighbouring number of children. After deliberation they coincidentally select same number.

Fertility decline is not the result of spread of a meme (R. Dawkins [17])—an idea, behavior, or style—from parents to parents within a given space. This realisation is not correct because it is difficult for RDE to spread the meme when we assume the meme of fertility decline. When an old meme which caused high fertility was the majority in a space, how can a new meme spread? Consequently we cannot help postulating the advantage or benefit of a new meme. Were there any benefit from the birth control in France around the end of eighteen century? A meme hypothesis cannot resolve these problems.

Another reason is that a meme is not well-defined so that we cannot verify its existence.

The final and simple consequence is that we act receiving the influence of neighbouring others. The most significant conception is that the way of receiving the influence of neighbouring others is universal.

2.2.2 Reaction as Disintegration of the Balance of Stochastic Fluctuations

The process of historical fertility decline suggests that there are a very few parents who acceleratingly diminish their number of children in reaction to the number of children in their space.

The reason of this reaction is explained by "disintegration of the balance of stochastic fluctuations". We may postulate following corollary to explain "Reaction".

Corollary 2.1 (Reaction as Outlier in Neighbourhood) *Parents rarely bear much different number of children from neighbourhood.*

Proposition 2.1 naturally includes this corollary. Also nowadays these rare numbers of children occur in lower and higher directions.[2] Before fertility decline, these rare

---

[2]These occurrences are also supported empirically. Even Hutterites have a maximum, a minimum, a mean, and a variances of their number of children.

occurrences balanced with each other. Statistically the average of the number of children is relatively stable then.

Corollary 2.2 (Reaction to One-way as declining fertility) *Child bearing is a product of behaviours more than two persons (a set of parents), whereas family limitation is not. The balance of each other inclines to disintegrated to lower directions.*

So the number of children of parents inclines to decline, if there are significant declines in neighbourhood. Let β be a highest fertility. $\beta - c(x)$ is a intensity of disintegration of balance. Let γ be a lowest fertility. $\gamma - c(x)$ is a room of decline.

2.2.3 Fertility Decline Difference Equation

When $c(x_0, t_0)$ significantly declines, what takes place? As a due course of our postulation, some decline of $c(x_0, t_0)$ affects other neighbouring segments' $c(x_i)$ recursively. Parents in each segment refer to each other, so at the next time period fertility in neighbouring segments' $c(x_{0-1}, t_1)$, $c(x_{0+1}, t_1)$ begins to decline. We can express this process in the following difference equation about $c(x_i, t_{k+1})$.

$$\begin{aligned} &c(x_i, t_{k+1}) \\ &\quad = \mu\, c(x_{i-1}, t_k) + \mu\, c(x_{i+1}, t_k) + \\ &\qquad (1 - 2\mu) \left[(c(x_i, t_k) + \alpha(\beta - c(x_i, t_k))(\gamma - c(x_i, t_k)) \right] \end{aligned} \tag{2.3}$$

μ is a coefficient of influence from adjoining segments. We can interpret it to be a coefficient of diffusion. We assume $0.0 \leq \mu \leq 1/2$. α is a coefficient of reaction within this $c(x_i)$ segment. Constant β is a highest fertility (=maximum $\overline{c}$). Constant γ is a lowest fertility (=minimum $\overline{c}$). Here after call Eq. (2.3) the **"Difference Equation of Spacial Distribution of Children (DESDC)"**. This difference equation is a reaction-diffusion system of the number of children in space.

When every $c(x_i, t_k) = \beta$, Eq. (2.3) is an equality (identity mapping). This state corresponds to maximum marital fertility. When every $c(x_i, t_k) = \gamma$, Eq. (2.3) is also an equality (identity mapping). This state corresponds to minimum marital fertility.

2.2.3.1 An Extreme Case of DESDC

We can think an undifferentiated space lacks neighbouring rectangles. The Eq. (2.3) degenerates to an equation of only the Reaction term.

$$c(x_i, t_{k+1}) = c(x_i, t_k) + \alpha(\beta - c(x_i, t_k))(\gamma - c(x_i, t_k) \tag{2.4}$$

This equation describes fertility decline in a macro scale population such as a nation-state. I name this equation MFDDE (Macro Fertility Decline Equation). I can obtain

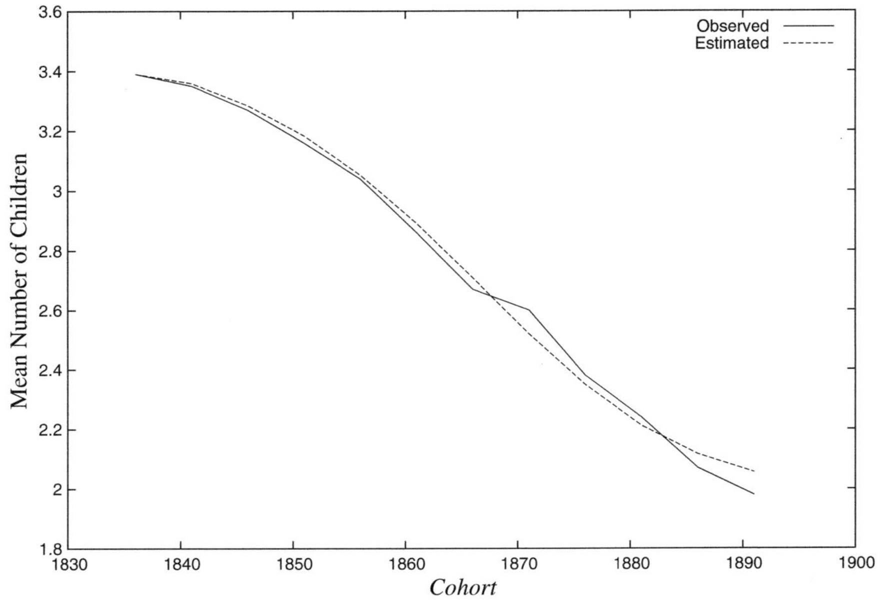

Fig. 2.2 Fertility decline of France and MFDDE. *Source* P. Festy [24], p. 48

fine fits of fertility decline for several European countries and Japan (Figs. 2.2, 2.3, 2.4, 2.5, 2.6).

These fine fits suggest that reaction-diffusion is a valid system to describe the fertility decline process of Europe and Japan (Table 2.1).

2.2.4 The Application of Fertility Decline Difference Equation

Next, I estimate coefficients μ, α from Japanese fertility decline processes, first with a space that is one dimensional and second with a two dimensional space.

2.2.4.1 One Dimensional Space

When we cut our geographical space from centre to periphery, we will observe one dimensional decline of fertility. By means of this linearisation, we can deal with our world as quasi-one dimensional one. It facilitates estimating coefficients μ, α for one dimensional space.

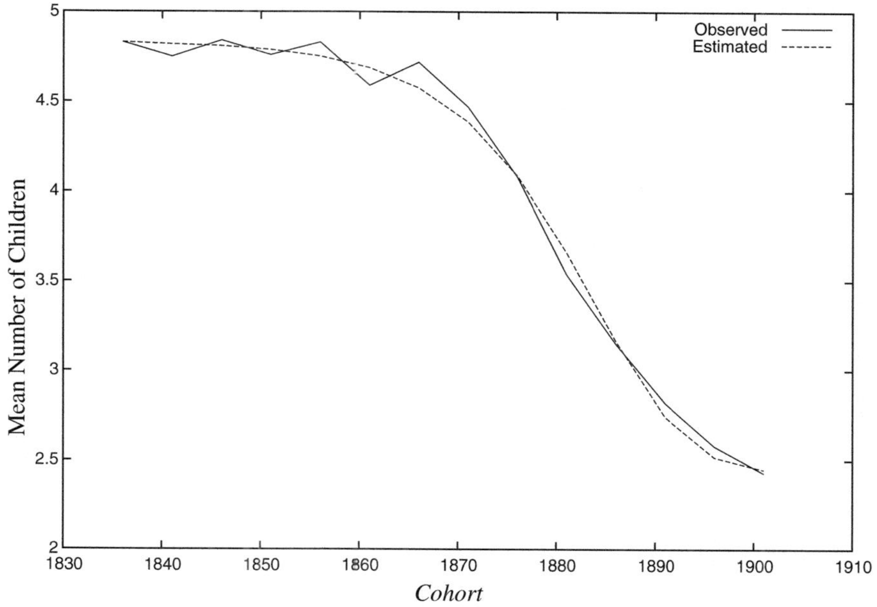

Fig. 2.3 Fertility decline of Finland and MFDDE. *Source* P. Festy [24], p. 48

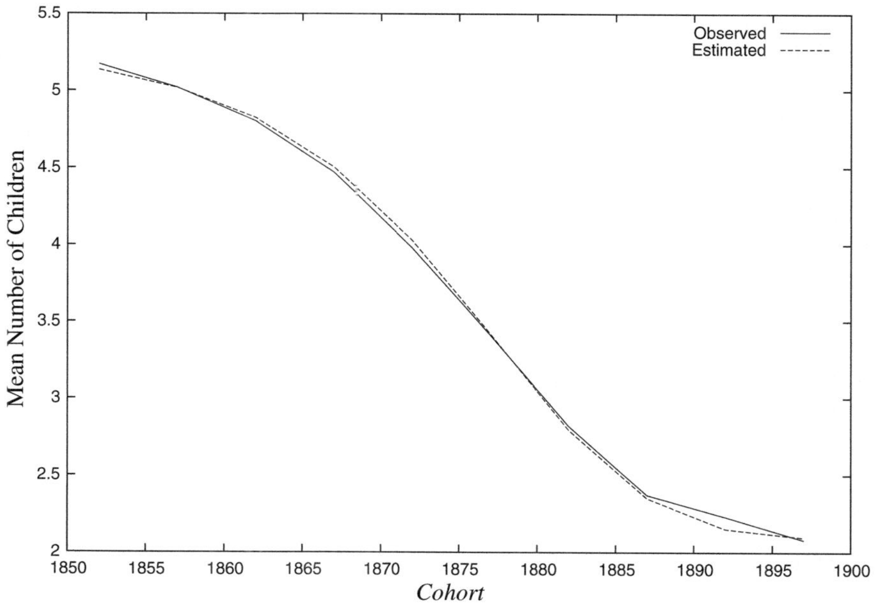

Fig. 2.4 Fertility decline of Germany and MFDDE. *Source* P. Festy [24], p. 49

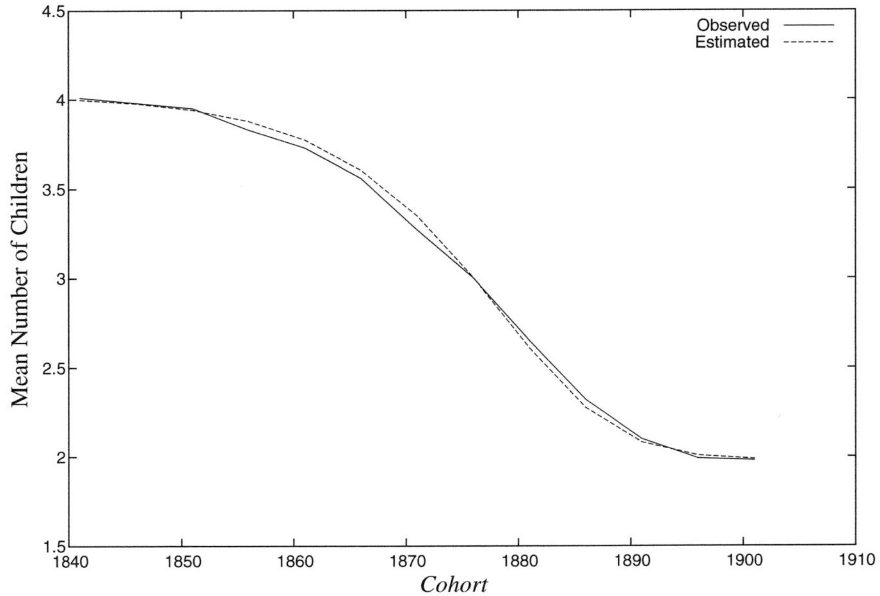

Fig. 2.5 Fertility decline of Swiss and MFDDE. *Source* P. Festy [24], p. 49

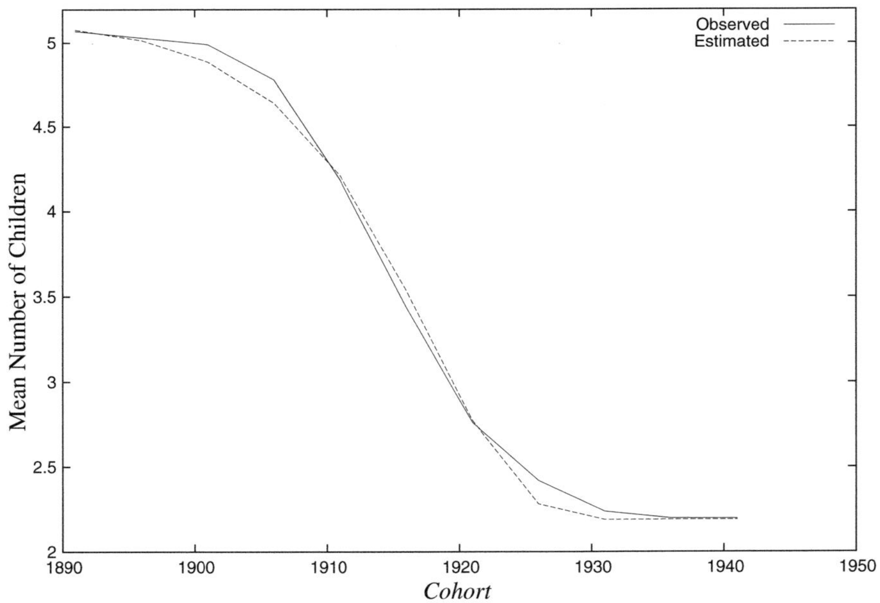

Fig. 2.6 Fertility decline of Japan and MFDDE. *Source* S. Ike [30], p. 38

Table 2.1 Estimated α', β, γ in MFDDE

	α'	β	γ	$\sum error^2$	Period
Japan	0.33376	5.146	2.11	0.066	1890–1940
France	0.31376	3.531	1.98	0.020	1836–1891
Finland	0.34414	4.833	2.43	0.075	1836–1901
Germany	0.25000	5.285	2.08	0.013	1852–1897
Swiss	0.37500	4.026	1.98	0.017	1841–1901

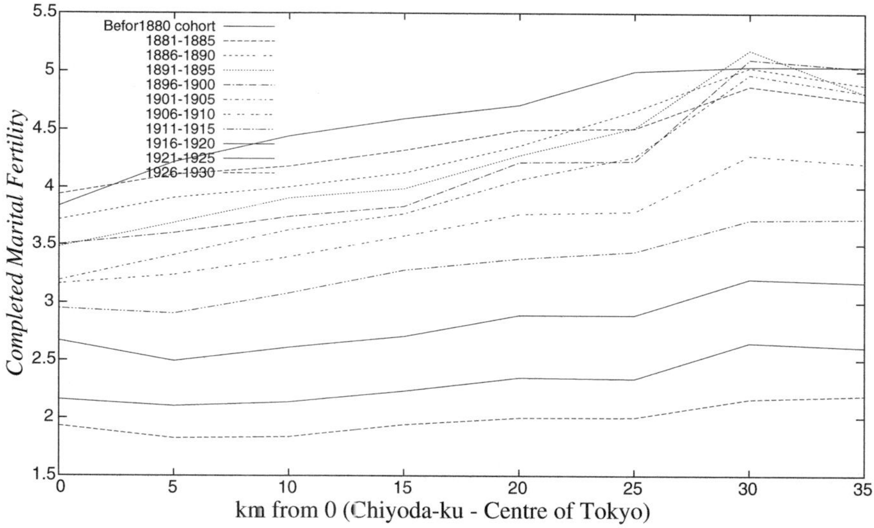

Fig. 2.7 Geographical marital fertility decline diffusion for Tokyo area. (observed). *Source* Sourihu Toukei Kyouku [62]

Thus I draw the following figures of geographical marital fertility decline diffusion for Tokyo area from Japanese census data (Fig. 2.7).[3]

The Method to Estimate μ, α

I use "direct search methods" [56] to find the estimations of μ, α. The direct search methods are those to find a minimizer (or maximizer) only by the values of functions, so it does not depend on Taylor expansion but on convex analysis. "Nelder-Mead

[3]Actually I selected Tokyo (the capital of Japan) area and Osaka (the centre of west Japan) and their surroundings. Japanese census recoded the means of number of children ever born of ever married women at 1960 and at 1970 by five-year cohorts for city, town and village. I draw circles with each radius (5, 10, 15, 20, 25, 30, 35 km) from the centre where fertility decline began. And I select some cities or towns or villages nearest to each circumference. I set an average of these $\overline{c}$ for a representative $\overline{c}_i$ at each radius. From 1896–1900 (born) cohort to 1921–1925 cohort, $c(x_i, t_k)$ was recoded for each cities.

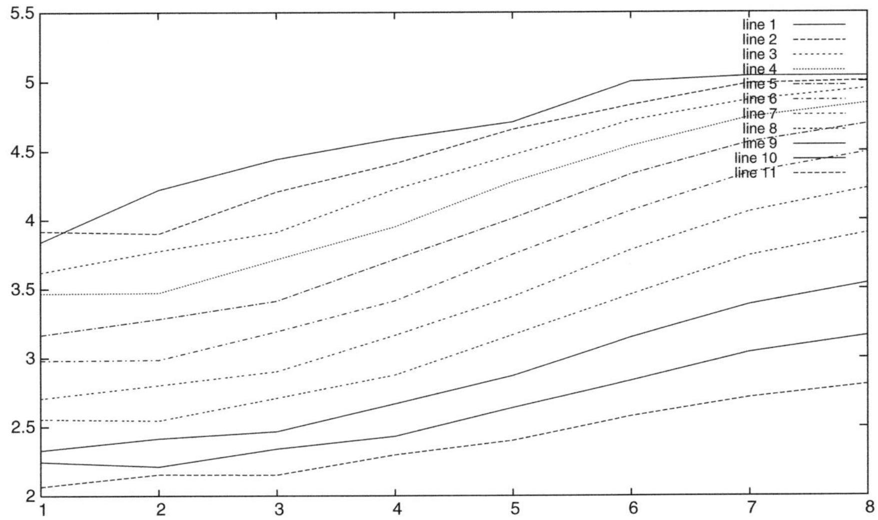

Fig. 2.8 Geographical marital fertility decline diffusion for Tokyo area. (estimated) $\mu = 0.4777, \alpha = 2.747, \beta = 5.11, \gamma = 2.11$. *line 1 = Before 1880 cohort, line 2 = 1881–1885, line 3 = 1886–1890, line 4 = 1891–1895, line 5 = 1896–1900, line 6 = 1901–1905, line 7 = 1906–1910, line 8 = 1911–1915, line 9 = 1916–1920, line 10 = 1921–1925, line 11 = 1926–1930

Simplex method" [18, 67] is the most frequently applied direct search method. This simplex method is robust against noises in function values and useful for problems of low dimensional variables. However it may not converge to a true minimizer and there is no adequate analysis of convergence.

I apply this Nelder-Mead Simplex method and subsidiary original algorithm (simulated annealing method [56]) to search for the minimizer by procedures to branch separated local space and search narrower area iteratively. This algorithm lacks the analytic bases. Unfortunately Nelder-Mead Simplex method depends upon the choice of the initial simplex, so several local minimizers are found with very slight difference of the sum of squares of residuals.

Nonetheless the simplex method can find a plausible minimiser for DESDC. Simplex method and simulated annealing method can find very approximate minimizers for μ, α (observed values are set for β, γ).

Next I draw the estimated figure of geographical marital fertility decline diffusion for Tokyo area (Fig. 2.8).

The DESDC can describe the geographical fertility reaction-diffusion process of Tokyo area in Japan fairly well (Table 2.2).

Table 2.2 Estimated μ, α, of Tokyo area

Method of estimation	μ	α	$\sum e^2$
Nelder-Mead simplex method (2)	0.47815	2.80000	3.73783
Simulated annealing method	0.47773	2.74658	3.74058

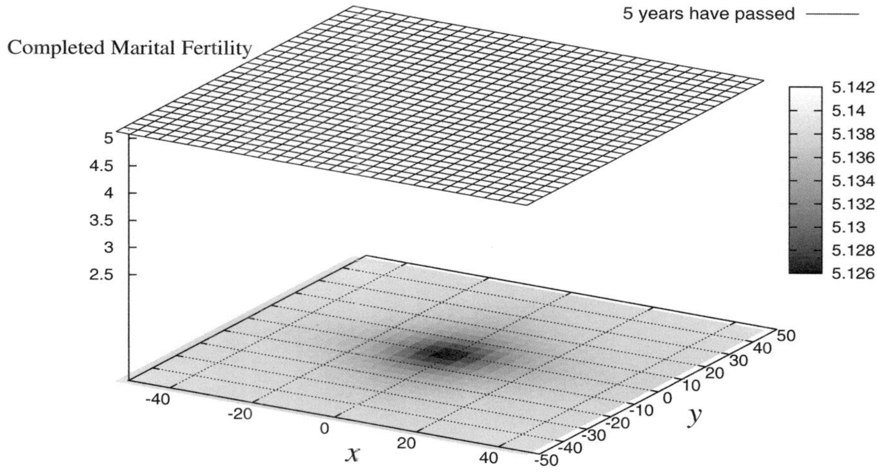

Fig. 2.9 Reaction-diffusion of fertility decline on two dimensional space (5 years have passed)

2.2.4.2 Two Dimensional Space

We can further extend DESDC to the equation for two dimensional space. Assume three dimensional surface composed by each rectangle $c(x_i, y_j)$. Let c be a mean number of children of each rectangle. A rectangle (x_i, y_j) correspond to geographical surface. c is imaged as a height of rectangle in three dimensional space. c is a function of x, y, t namely of space-time.

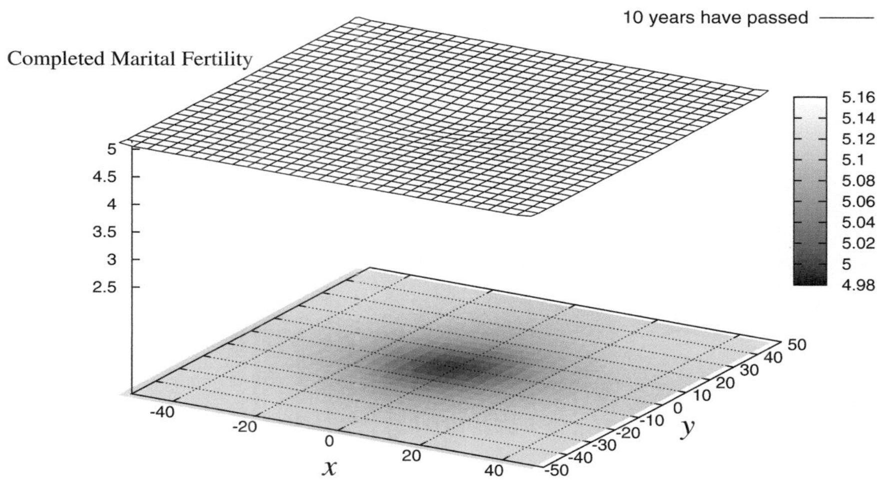

Fig. 2.10 Reaction-diffusion of fertility decline on two dimensional space (10 years have passed)

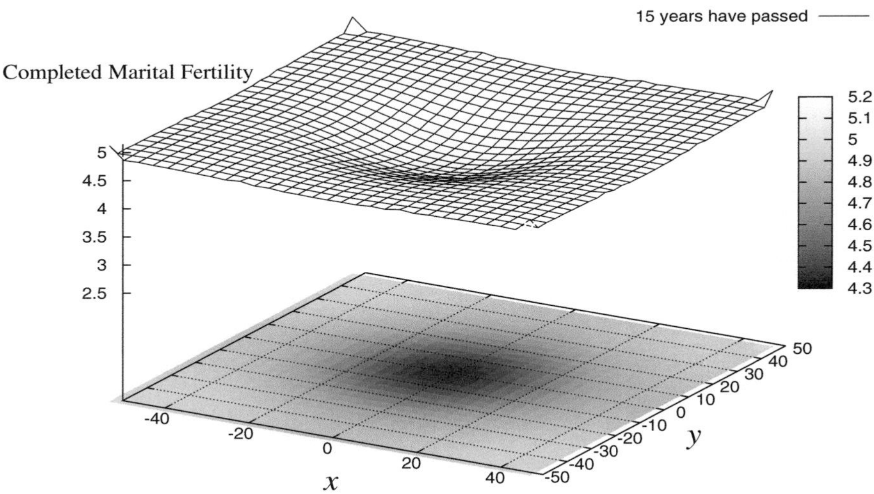

Fig. 2.11 Reaction-diffusion of fertility decline on two dimensional space (15 years have passed)

Consider a population distributed in a two dimensional space with c surface. Let $c(x_i, y_j, t_k)$ be a mean of the number of children of rectangle (x_i, y_j) at time k. Let $c(x_{i-1}, y_j, t_k)$, $c(x_{i+1}, y_j, t_k)$, $c(x_i, y_{j-1}, t_k)$, $c(x_i, y_{j+1}, t_k)$ be a mean of the number of children of neighbouring rectangles at time t_k.

From isotropy of Proposition 2.1, neighbouring rectangles $c(x_i, y_j, t_k)$ equally affect each other. Therefore $c(x_i, y_j, t_{k+1})$ is expressed from $c(x_{i-1}, y_j, t_k)$, $c(x_{i+1}, y_j, t_k)$, $c(x_i, y_j, t_k)$, $c(x_i, y_{j-1}, t_k)$, $c(x_i, y_{j+1}, t_k)$ as the following difference equation (Figs. 2.9 and 2.10).

$$\begin{aligned} & c(x_i, y_j, t_{k+1}) \\ & = \mu\, c(x_{i-1}, y_j, t_k) + \mu\, c(x_{i+1}, y_j, t_k) + \\ & \quad \mu\, c(x_i, y_{j-1}, t_k) + \mu\, c(x_i, y_{j+1}, t_k) + \\ & \quad (1 - 4\mu) \left[c(x_i, y_j, t_k) + \alpha(\beta - c(x_i, y_j, t_k))(\gamma - c(x_i, y_j, t_k)) \right] \end{aligned} \tag{2.5}$$

If at an origin, at $t = 0$, $c(x_0, y_0, t_0)$ declines significantly, neighbouring $c(x_i, y_j, t_1)$ begins to decline recursively by the Difference Equation DESDC (2.5) from origin to peripheral rectangles. We image a process of fertility decline as a developing hole in 3D surface like Fig. 2.11. For two dimensional space, we can also numerically simulate a reaction-diffusion system.

2.2.5 Differential Equation of Fertility Decline

By Taylor expansion, difference equation DESDC (2.5) is transposed to a differential equation. This conversion allows examining the velocity of the diffusion wave from the differential equation of spacial distribution of children (SDC) (Fig. 2.12).

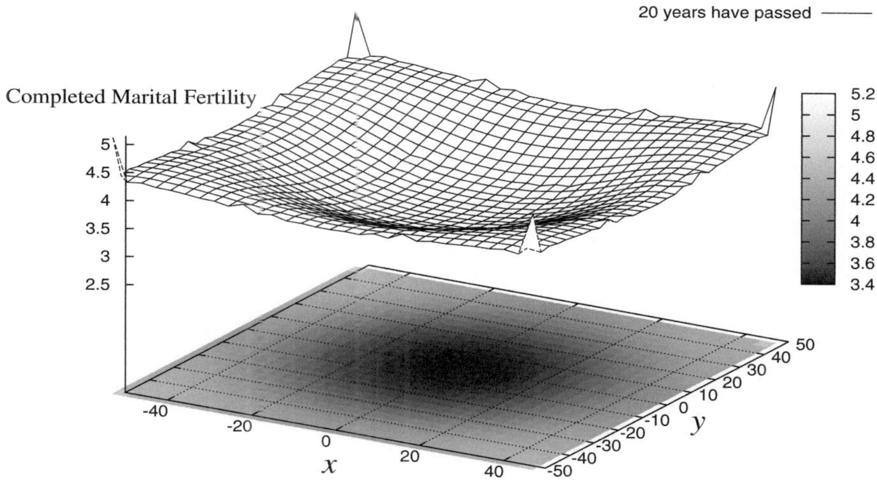

Fig. 2.12 Reaction-diffusion of fertility decline on two dimensional space (20 years have passed)

$$\frac{\partial c(x, y, t)}{\partial t} = \mu \frac{\partial^2 c(x, y, t)}{\partial x^2} \frac{\Delta a^2}{\Delta t} + \mu \frac{\partial^2 c(x, y, t)}{\partial y^2} \frac{\Delta a^2}{\Delta t} + \frac{(1 - 4\mu)}{\Delta t} \alpha(\beta - c(x, y, t))(\gamma - c(x, y, t)) \quad (2.6)$$

When we accept a relation $\Delta a^2 = \Delta t = (1 - 4\mu)$ in an infinite transportation, differential equation (2.6)

$$\frac{\partial c(x, y, t)}{\partial t} = \mu \frac{\partial^2 c(x, y, t)}{\partial x^2} + \mu \frac{\partial^2 c(x, y, t)}{\partial y^2} + \alpha(\beta - c(x, y, t))(\gamma - c(x, y, t)) \quad (2.7)$$

turn to the equation above with the same coefficients as the difference equation DESDC. This procedure means that we minimise rectangles to a limit of space-time.

We can write this differential equation using two dimensional value c and Laplacian Δ in another style as following.

$$\frac{\partial c}{\partial t} = \mu \Delta c + \alpha(\beta - c)(\gamma - c) \quad (2.8)$$

2.2.5.1 Variances of Fertility Decline Are Proportional to Time in Its Initial Stage

As long as the effects of Reaction-term are still little, we can recognise the differential equation (2.7) as a normal diffusion equation. We obtain an analytical basic solution as the Eq. (2.9).

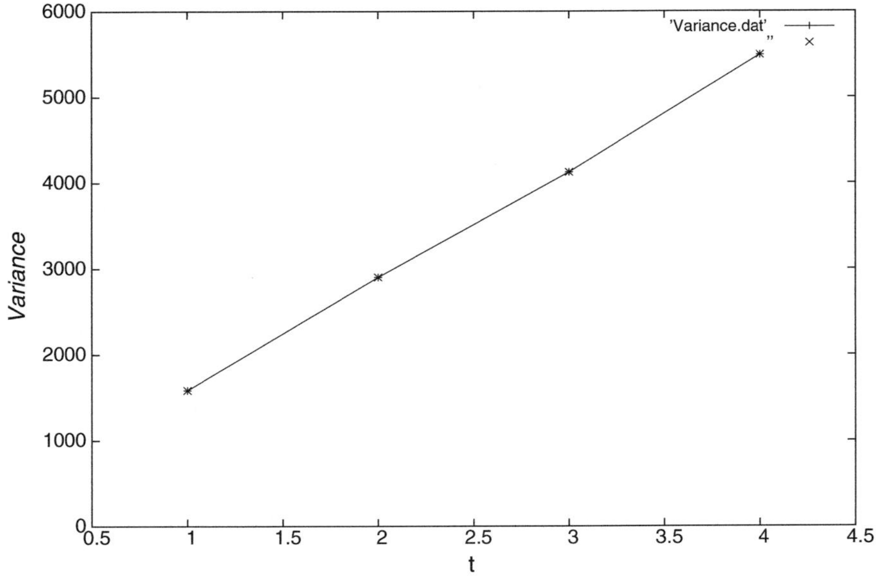

Fig. 2.13 Variances of fertility decline with time t in Hokaido

$$f(x,t) = \frac{1}{\sqrt{4\pi t}} \exp\left(-\frac{x^2}{4t}\right) \tag{2.9}$$

It is just a normal distribution. We can find a relation $2t = \sigma^2$ in this equation. When fertility decline is described by the differential equation (2.7), variances of the amount of fertility decline are proportional to time t.

I have already observed fertility decline processes of three areas in Japan. All three areas Hokkaido, Tokyo, and Osaka have been observed over 50 years and their data of variances of fertility decline in initial 20 years analyzed. All these three areas showed a very similar upward tendency. However, the proportionality in Tokyo and Osaka cases seemed a bit imperfect. The linearity in Hokkaido was almost perfect (Fig. 2.13). [4, 5]

[4]I believe this is because of the size of the area that data cover, with Tokyo and Osaka being much smaller regions than Hokkaido. In order to demonstrate the perfect proportionality, in line with the argument by J.G. Skellam I have resorted to use Hokkaido case, roughly 9 times as large as those in Tokyo, Osaka.

[5]The famous article in mathematical ecology by J.G. Skellam [61] reported the same linearity of diffusion of muskrats from Bohemia to mid-Europe. In his article, the space is widened from Munich to Breslau—in a circle with 300 km radius.

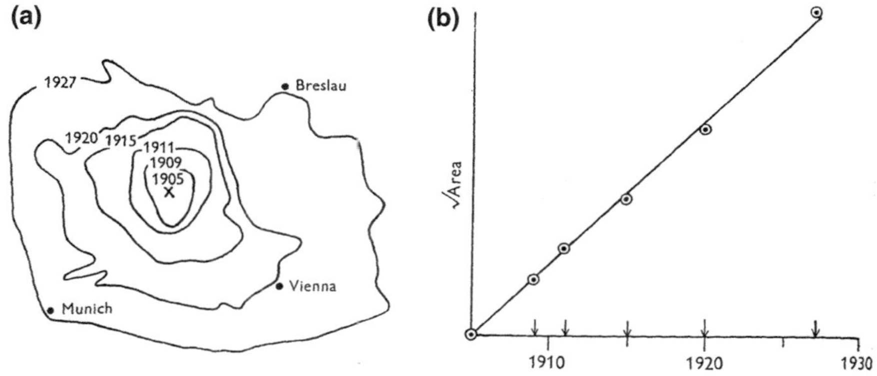

Fig. 2.14 The Spread of the muskrat—**a** The apparent boundaries, **b** The relation between time and $\sqrt{}$area. *Source* J. G. Skellam [61], p. 200

2.2.5.2 Properties of Reaction-Diffusion Equation of Fertility Decline

A nontrivial solution of the differential equation SDC (2.7) has some properties that is specifically observed in the phenomena of fertility decline. A solution of reaction-diffusion equation has a remarkable effect of smoothing (even though it depends on the balance of coefficients μ and α).

This smoothing effect explains the irreversibility, stability, and smoothing of fertility decline. After "demographic transition", except for baby boom, fertility in developed countries have not risen up again. Baby boom was terminated at last and marital fertility have been converging to the minimum level of fertility in the developed countries. Marital fertility of them has been rather stable. Since smoothing effects have governed each parents in space-time, differences of fertility could had been brought about by socio-economic status have been diminishing. In other words, neighbouring dependency of the number of children of parents is an essential element. Differential fertility observed in the past was a temporal phenomenon caused by a partial geographical distribution of socio-economic status.

2.2.6 Progressive Wave

A nontrivial solution of the differential equation SDC (2.7) is called a "Kolmogoroff-Pertrovsky-Piscounoff Progressive Wave" [43] (Fig. 2.14).

It is drawn graphically in Fig. 2.15. Progressive wave spread from a singularity to peripherals. In time the points where minimum fertility decline occurred had advanced to peripherals. We call these points "front" or "edge" of Progressive Wave (See "*Front*" in Fig. 2.15). In other words, when front arrives, fertility decline begins.

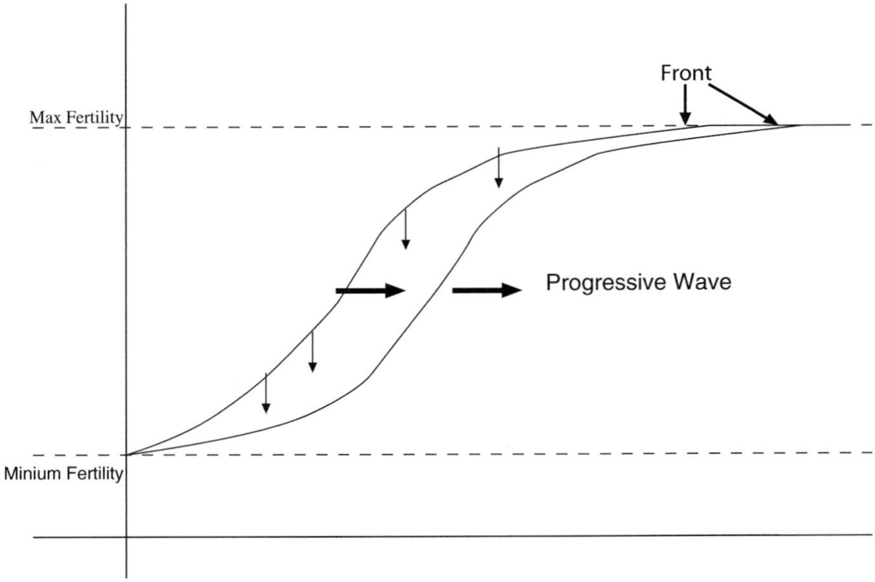

Fig. 2.15 Progressive wave of fertility decline

2.2.6.1 The Velocity for One Dimensional Space

R.A. Fisher [25] showed this progressive wave has a velocity. His mathematical model is designed for one dimensional space. This low dimensionality is rather convenient for our purpose of estimation.

For each geographical point, the times the front of wave takes to arrive differs proportional to the distances from a singularity. Thus by means of the difference in time when marital fertility decline began we are able to estimate the velocity of progressive wave.

For Japan, I estimate $10\,\text{km/year} \le v \le 14\,\text{km/year}$ as the velocity of the front of wave from differences of the occurrence of fertility decline in time recorded in census data is shown Table 2.3.

On the other hand, we previously obtained the estimations of μ, α by Simplex method. Fisher deduced that $v = 2\sqrt{\mu\alpha}$ in one dimensional space. In order to be accord the observations with a unit of velocity (km per year) in our data to, it is necessary to multiply the intervals of the ratio of the square of space (h^2) and to divide the ratio of time (k) to each coefficient. The data which I employ to estimate them are composed of means of children for segments (5 km long) by 5 years. So I multiply $\mu\alpha$ by $\frac{h^4}{k^2}$. Therefore the velocity of progressive wave of fertility decline (unit km per year) is calculated by the following expression.

Table 2.3 Distance and time progressive wave (front) took to arrive in Japan

From	Arrived area	Distance	Passed time	Estimated velocity
Tokyo	Marginal Kanto area	(max) 50 km	< 5 year	10 km/year >
Tokyo	Niigata	270 km	From 20 to 25 years	From 10.5 to 13.5 km/year
Sapporo	Hokaido	(max) 140 km	in 10 years	14 km/year

Kanto is the name of zone around Tokyo. Tokyo is one of the singularities of fertility decline in Japan. Niigata is the biggest of the cities front on the Japan Sea. Tokyo is the city fronts on Pacific Ocean, namely progressive wave ran cross the Japanese Island. Sapporo is the centre of Hokaido which is an isolated island of north Japan

$$2\sqrt{\mu\alpha}\,\frac{h^2}{k} \tag{2.10}$$

I substitute the previously obtained estimations (Table 2.2) for each μ, α in the expression (2.10). Thus I calculate an estimation of velocity (km per year) of progressive wave as a following expression.

$$11.45 < 2\sqrt{\mu\alpha}\,\frac{5^2}{5} < 11.68$$

These estimations resemble the values obtained by differences of time and distances between two points where fertility decline occurred. This resemblance supports the validity of a difference equation DESDC.

2.2.6.2 The Velocity for Two Dimensional Space

The velocity of wave in two dimensional space is $\sqrt{2\mu\alpha}$. Namely the front of wave moves with velocity $\sqrt{2\mu\alpha}$ in our surface. I obtained estimations of μ, α for two dimensional space composed of 1 km^2 rectangles by one month.

Therefore the velocity of progressive wave of fertility decline (unit km per year) for two dimensional space is calculated by the following expression.

$$\sqrt{2\mu\alpha}\,\frac{h^2}{k} \tag{2.11}$$

The estimations are somewhat smaller than those for one dimensional space.

$$10.04 < \sqrt{2\mu\alpha}\,\frac{1^2}{\frac{1}{12}} < 10.67$$

However this resemblance of estimations between one dimension and two dimensions suggests the validity of two difference equations.

2.3 A Search for a Singularity-Origin of Fertility Decline in Europe

In differential equation (2.8), when we go back to time $t = 0$,

$$\lim t \to 0, \quad \frac{\partial c}{\partial t} = \mu \Delta c + \alpha(\beta - c)(\gamma - c) \to 0 \tag{2.12}$$

a partial differentiation is infinitely small. We must postulate a quantum of decline of c at time $t = 0$. This point is a singularity, in other words an origin of fertility decline.

By means of the estimated velocity of progressive wave of fertility decline, we are able to determine when and where a singularity of fertility decline was in Europe.

First of all, since France is the first country which began fertility decline, a singularity must exist in France. The question which should be solved is that in which district of France the singularity of fertility decline was.

2.3.1 The Date When a Singularity Appeared

The key is differences in time between countries when fertility decline began. From isomorphism of progressive wave, the differences between dates of decline by 10 % is nearly equal to the differences between dates of the beginning of fertility decline.

Then I obtain the differences in time by 10 % about some countries as in Table 2.4. These differences correspond to the differences in time when the minimum fertility decline began.

This means that when we know the date of the beginning of fertility decline in Germany and other places, we can estimate the time of the occurrence of a singularity in France. So I examine the dates when fertility decline began in European countries (Table 2.5).

In Germany 1852–1860 cohort began to decline its fertility. In Denmark 1855–1859. In Belgium 1836–1845. In Netherlands 1851–1860. We can calculate the date when a singularity occur by simple subtractions. For example $1852 - 90 = 1762$ for Germany. I suppose a singularity appeared in cohort born between 1754 and 1772.

Table 2.4 Date of decline in marital fertility by 10 %

France	Germany	Denmark	Belgium	Netherlands
ca. 1800	1890	1900	1882	1897

Source J. Knodel and Etienne van de Walle [36], pp. 221–222

Table 2.5 Initial fertility decline of Germany, Denmark, Belgium, and Netherlands

Germany		Denmark		Belgium		Netherlands	
Cohort	CTFR	Cohort	CTFR	Cohort	CTFR	Cohort	CTFR
1852–1860	5.17	1840–1844	4.39	**1836–1845**	4.50	1836–1845	5.06
1857–1865	5.02	1845–1849	4.41	1841–1850	4.43	1841–1850	5.13
1862–1870	4.80	1850–1854	4.44	1846–1855	4.30	1846–1855	5.16
		1855–1859	4.38			**1851–1860**	4.98
		1860–1864	4.16			1856–1865	4.64

Source Fertility in Western Countries from 1870 to 1970, pp. 48–49, [24].

It is plausible that a singularity appeared in a last half of 1750s cohort, so it occurred about in 1770s in France as real period date.

2.3.2 *Where Is a Singularity?*

If we make an assumption that a velocity of progressive wave is universally equal about 10 km/year, we are able to determine the location of the singularity. It took almost 90 years for progressive wave to arrive to Germany from a singularity. This means that the singularity is about 900 km away from Germany. It took 82 years for progressive wave to arrive to Belgium so the singularity is about 820 km away from Belgium.

I let Frankfurt am Main be a representative point for Germany (Frankfurt was near the then centre of population gravity of Germany.) and Brussels for Belgium. I drew a circle which has a centre of Frankfurt and a radius of 900 km.[6] I also drew a circle which has a centre of Brussels and a radius of 820 km. One of the intersections of the circles is the point that a singularity of fertility decline appeared. Namely the estimated point is around *Aquitaine* district (Fig. 2.16).

2.3.2.1 Lot-et-Garonne

After I estimated *Aquitaine* as a singularity, I noticed somehow incidentally the critical fact. A proceeding study recorded that Lot-et-Garonne in *Aquitaine* had the lowest fertility in Europe. A.J. Coale and R.Treadway [13] pointed out that the French *département* of Lot-et-Garonne was the bottom of marital fertility in Europe.

[6] If we set Hamburg as a point to draw a circle, as Hamburg started fertility decline around 1880 (from *Coale and Treadway* [13]), it took about 110 years to arrive, so we drew a radius of 1100 km. The intersection is still on *Aquitaine*.

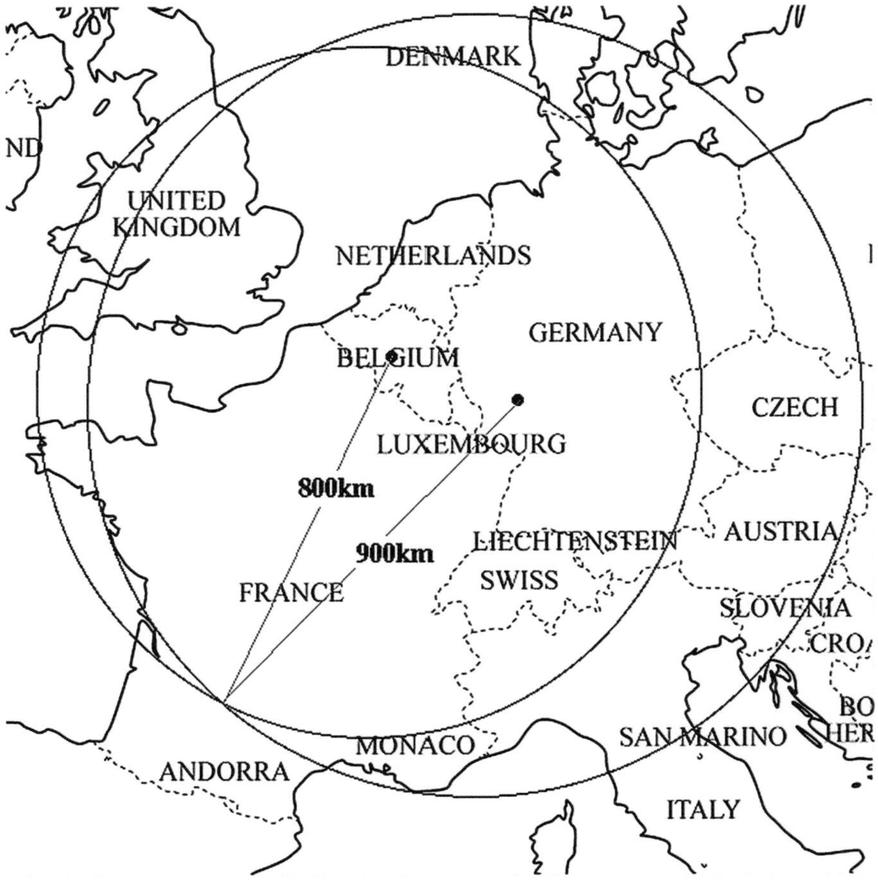

Fig. 2.16 The point 900 km from Frankfurt am Main and 800 km from Brussels

A sense of the meaning of these indexes can be gained by considering some examples. Three provinces at the bottom of the range (the lowest 10 % in the distribution) of overall fertility (I_f) in Europe in 1900 were **Lot-et-Garonne** (a *département* of France), Geneva, and County Tipperary in Ireland. The overall rate of childbearing in the first two areas was only about one-sixth of the Hutterites (I_f of 0.168 and 0.164), while in Tipperary I_f was a little higher at 0.220.

Ansley J. Coale and Roy Treadway [13], p. 34 (boldfaced by author)

The French *départment* of Lot-et-Garonne had especially low fertility from a very early date, and the age distribution of women in 1900 from 15 to 50 was nearly uniform. I_m in Lot-et-Garonne (0.700) was the highest in Western Europe; with the age distribution of Russia it would have been 0.699. Without the special age distribution generated by its history of especially low fertility, the I_m of of Lot-et-Garonne would still have been highest (or nealy so) in Western Europe.

Ansley J. Coale and Roy Treadway [13], p. 159

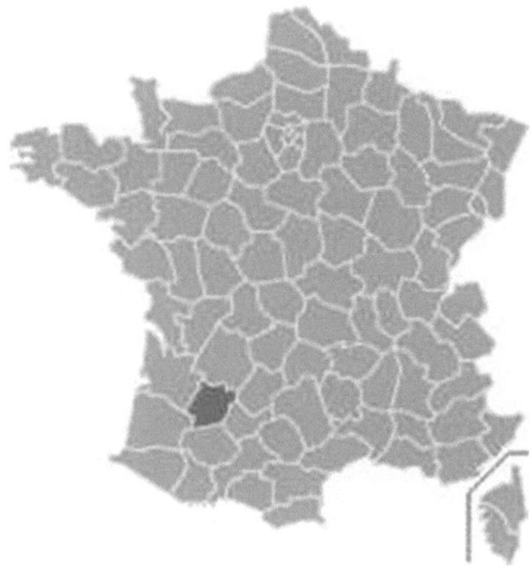

Fig. 2.17 Geographical location of Lot-et-Garonne. *Source* http://fr.wikipedia.org/wiki/Lot-et-Garonne April, 30, 2015

There is a relation between I_f and I_m, I_g that $I_f \simeq I_m \cdot I_g$. So the marital fertility of Lot-et-Garonne is the lowest in western Europe.[7] In 1831 $I_g = 0.351$ is estimated for Lot-et-Garonne. These data means that Lot-et-Garonne was the lowest of marital fertility in western Europe.

Therefore I speculate that a singularity is *département* of Lot-et-Garonne in *Aquitaine*. This coincidence that the point of the lowest fertility existed in *Aquitaine* suggests that coefficients μ, α are universal constants and that reaction-diffusion exactly traces the fertility decline process in Europe.

2.3.2.2 Why Lot-et-Garonne Not Paris?

Economic growth definitely increases fertility as "Easterlin Hypothesis" [19–21]. If a singularity might have occurred near London, economic growth caused by industrialisation filled up the singularity before it developed. Economic growth is an interference with fertility decline (Fig. 2.17).

The confusion created by the French Revolution could have robbed a singularity of its diffusion mechanism. A singularity had to come into existence in the point far from "Industrialisation" and "Revolutions". This coincidence was amazing and providential.

---

[7] Geneva's I_g was 0.458 in 1860. This figure is far more than Lot-et-Garonne. Low fertility of Geneva was caused by the low level of I_m—low level of the rate of ever married. Swiss still remained in the medieval fertility control stage.

2.3.2.3 The Probability of Disintegration of the Balance

The questions why no singularities in centuries before 1770, and why no singularities in Sweden or Italy are natural and intelligent. I try to give an answer to them.

I think that the singularity is equal to the decisive disintegration of the balance of stochastic fluctuations of the number of children in the direction to declining the number of children. Even though the appearance of the singularity is a genuine coincidence, the probability that it appears is absolutely small. So it takes a long time for the decisive disintegration of the balance of stochastic fluctuations to occur.

I calculate its probability experimentally. Medieval villages had 400–450 population on average consisting of about 50 families. Suppose that the size of the singularity is a village, the occurrence of a singularity requires that completed marital fertility must continuously decline for ten or twenty years without any socio-economic disturbance.

The probability that all neighbouring 30 or 35 sets of parents (they are neighbouring in the time axis) simultaneously decline their completed fertility is roughly calculated at $10^{-3} \sim 3.64 \times 10^{-5}$ per year. This is the reason that the singularity had not occurred before 1770.

I cannot know the minimum size of singularity, therefore this probability could be smaller or larger. I think the occurrence is a lucky coincident which may take place once or not once for previous human history. This is an answer why the singularity had not occurred before.

I will also give an answer to the other question why the singularity occurred in France not in Sweden or Italy or others. I think that the answer is also a genuine coincidence. However the probability of disintegration of the balance of stochastic fluctuations was higher in *Lot-et-Garonne* than other places. Its marriage rate was known to be the highest of all Europe. In addition to it, political, economic and social conditions were quite stable. These higher uniformity of the major sets of parents in *Lot-et-Garonne* prompted the disintegration. The high uniformity inclines to break spontaneously.

2.4 Reaction-Diffusion from the Singularity of Lot-et-Garonne

The early diffusionists recorded the province-wise process of fertility decline in Europe. The reaction-diffusion model is constructed based on the number of children in the space, because the number of children in the space lattice width facilitates an examination of the model's its validity.[8]

[8]Strictly speaking, smaller is not better. There is a lower limit of the space lattice and time pitch widths when the numbers of children of each set of parents are treated in a stochastic manner. Of course these widths are much larger within statistical data.

The data collected for the Princeton European Fertility Project from the 1960s to the 1970s is invaluable. The findings of this project were published as a book entitled, *The Decline of Fertility in Europe*, edited by Coale and Watkins. Using these data, I will trace the reaction-diffusion process based on each province's I_g (index of marital fertility, for the definition, see p. 15.), as recorded in *The Decline of Fertility in Europe*.

Mainland France is currently composed of 95 départments. However, it should be noted that these départments are not the same as those investigated by Coale and the early diffusionists. Based on institutional transitions that occurred, I will first estimate a singularity (the origin of fertility decline). I will then examine peripheral areas of the singularity in central France and the départments that were last to experience fertility decline (Fig. 2.18).

Although early diffusionists such as Coale and Treadway frequently referred to Lot-et-Garonne as having the lowest fertility, they did not conceive of it as an origin

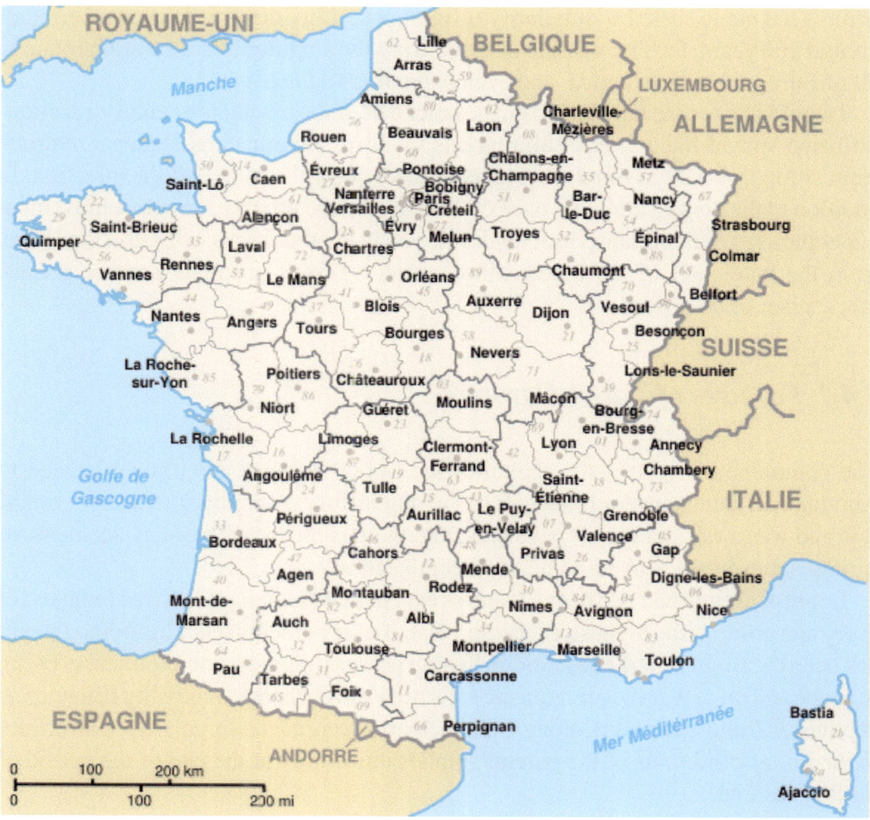

Fig. 2.18 Préfectures de France. *Source* http://ja.wikipedia.org/wiki/2eAu:Préfectures_de_France.svg

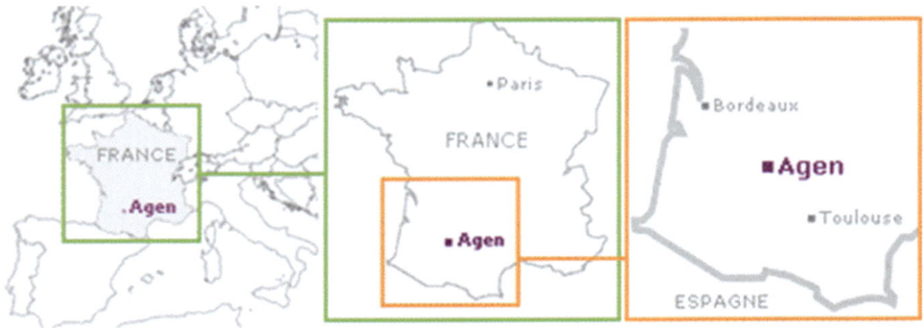

Fig. 2.19 The location of Agen in Lot-et-Garonne. *Source* http://www.agen.fr/1-12516-Situation-acces.php

point of the fertility decline in Europe. Because they did not use a mathematical model of diffusion to investigate the process of fertility decline, they could not perceive an origin point for its diffusion.

My examination of spatial variation of the number of children for each set of parents led me to seek the singularity (origin) of fertility decline. During a period of around 200 years, fertility decline diffused from the singularity at Lot-et-Garonne to all of Europe, North America, and even extending to East Asia.

I would like to note here that from the latter half of the nineteenth century, reaction-diffusion spread like wildfire. Immigrants in North America and students returned from abroad, as well as hired foreigners in Japan were the source of the infection. In addition to the normal crawling pace of diffusion on the ground, the active movement of people as a result of transportation development altered the pace of diffusion. Thus, from the latter half of the nineteenth century, we must postulate another precise mechanism of diffusion.

2.4.1 Features of Lot-et-Garonne

The commune of Agen is the capital of the Lot-et-Garonne département located in Aquitaine in southwestern France. It has a long history dating back to ancient times. It is and was a relaxed countryside area, and there is no mention of any accidents or significant events occurring in the eighteenth century (Fig. 2.19).

Lot-et-Garonne had no special features except that the ratio of married females for every age group is the highest, exceeding that of every other place. This homogeneity has been the trigger for the reaction-diffusion process. Against common sense, living in peace and quiet was the prerequisite for a truly novel change of fertility behavior. A decline by Zufall[9] (fortuity), along with fluctuation caused the singularity. Uniformity in the initial conditions of the parents implies uniformity at the end of the period of fertility decline.

[9]"Kein Sieger glaubt an den Zufall." (F. Nietzsche) I think fertility decline in the European modern period was the coincidence.

Table 2.6 Changes in I_g in Lot-et-Garonne and neighboring *départments*

	Lot-et-Garonne	Gironde	Dordogne	Landes	Pyrenees-Atlantiques*	Gers	Lot	Tarn-et-Garonne	Corse
1831	0.351	0.393	0.520	0.624	0.621	0.421	0.509	0.390	0.683
1836	0.339	0.375	0.496	0.592	0.595	0.395	0.493	0.364	0.701
1841	0.333	0.358	0.472	0.585	0.597	0.380	0.486	0.351	0.681
1846	0.315	0.333	0.461	0.556	0.576	0.352	0.465	0.337	0.676
1851	0.298	0.341	0.452	0.562	0.563	0.338	0.446	0.329	0.656
1856	0.290	0.338	0.447	0.528	0.577	0.328	0.446	0.330	0.646
1861	0.282	0.336	0.451	0.511	0.580	0.321	0.437	0.328	0.636
1866	0.279	0.338	0.468	0.513	0.566	0.337	0.435	0.328	0.656
1871	0.280	0.316	0.465	0.534	0.589	0.346	0.429	0.325	0.676
1876	0.271	0.308	0.453	0.530	0.614	0.333	0.418	0.316	0.685
1881	0.266	0.303	0.437	0.506	0.622	0.316	0.385	0.299	0.710
1886	0.246	0.287	0.398	0.475	0.620	0.290	0.331	0.283	0.727
1891	0.232	0.265	0.371	0.440	0.601	0.259	0.319	0.274	0.710
1896	0.230	0.256	0.361	0.403	0.591	0.247	0.329	0.273	0.632
1901	0.230	0.245	0.352	0.392	0.576	0.241	0.333	0.274	0.593
1911	0.207	0.212	0.294	0.294	0.444	0.219	0.271	0.242	0.510
1921	0.240	0.256	0.307	0.291	0.414	0.254	0.296	0.282	0.479
1931	0.238	0.219	0.273	0.252	0.343	0.257	0.262	0.265	0.331
1961	0.288	0.283	0.279	0.304	0.348	0.302	0.310	0.306	0.508

Source Ansley J. Coale and Roy Treadway [13].
The recovery period commenced from 1921. The baby boom affected the I_g for 1961.
*Only Pyrenees-Atlantiques is not a direct neighbor of Lot-et-Garonne. This is the reason why the fertility decline effect of the singularity was relatively small for Pyrenees-Atlantiques

According to E. van de Walle, the level of fertility in Lot-et-Garonne was below the population replacement level. Consequently, from 1836, its population monotonically declined, even without emigration.[10] The reaction-diffusion process was propelled by its inertia and could not, therefore, stop until it reached its lower limit.

2.5 Areas Around the Singularity: Aquitaine and Parts of the Midi-Pyrénées

We can identify the $I_f, I_g, and I_m$ in all of the French provinces from 1830 by referring to *The Decline of Fertility in Europe*. For details on the I_g, see Table 2.6. The progressive wave traveled at 10 km per year from the singularity, and by 1831, the fertility of neighboring *départments* had already evidenced a natural decline.

[10] The commune of Agen did not disappear. It remains a beautiful garden city, as portrayed on the website http://www.agen/fr/ The decline of fertility did not endure.

Applying the reaction-diffusion hypothesis, I estimated that the singularity of fertility decline occurred for the 1750–1760 birth cohort. Consequently, the decline of I_g should have started during the period from 1770–1780. About 60 years should have passed from the occurrence of singularity in 1830.

Fertility decline began in 1836 in the island of Corsica (Corse Département). This date is reasonable given that the progressive wave from Cote D'Azur was obstructed by the Mediterranean Sea.

2.5.1 Background Independence of Fertility Decline

The French industrial revolution temporarily restrained the fertility decline. The temporariness of the ascent of fertility (I_g) strongly implies background independence of fertility decline.

2.5.1.1 Effects of Economic Development: Restraint Factors in Fertility Decline

Although by 1830, *départments* on the periphery of Lot-et-Garonne began to evident fertility decline, all of them had temporarily moved away from the monotonic locus of decline by around 1860. The rise in fertility at the singularity, namely, Lot-et-Garonne, and in neighboring Gironde was only slight. However, other *départments* recorded a significant ascent of I_g from 1860 to 1880.

This significant ascent was caused by the economic development that took place during the period of the Second French Empire under the reign of Napoleon III. During this period French industries grew at an extraordinary pace, resulting in the provision of ample employment. Construction of the railways and the remodeling of Paris during the reign of Napoleon III required a huge amount of manpower, and contributed to a rise of fertility. The evolving industrialization at that time demanded many workers. This same mechanism resulted in population growth in England and Wales during the early nineteenth century.

However this ascent was impermanent, because, as is always the case, economic development did not sustain. Even if this ascent of fertility by economic development was temporary, should inverse arising of fertility have occurred in the decline process under the constant dynamics of the decline caused by the reaction-diffusion system? We should note that the index I_g is the periodical index of fertility, and not for cohorts. When there was an inclination toward early marriage and early births, without any change in the completed fertility of cohorts, I_g increased, as reflected in numerical values. This estimation is supported by the phenomenon of an accelerated decline after the ascent (Fig. 2.20).

Of course at some points, the increase of completed marital fertility of each set of parents may occur. Indeed the French industrial revolution brought about a small baby boom, but as long as fertility was relatively low at the singularity, the fertility

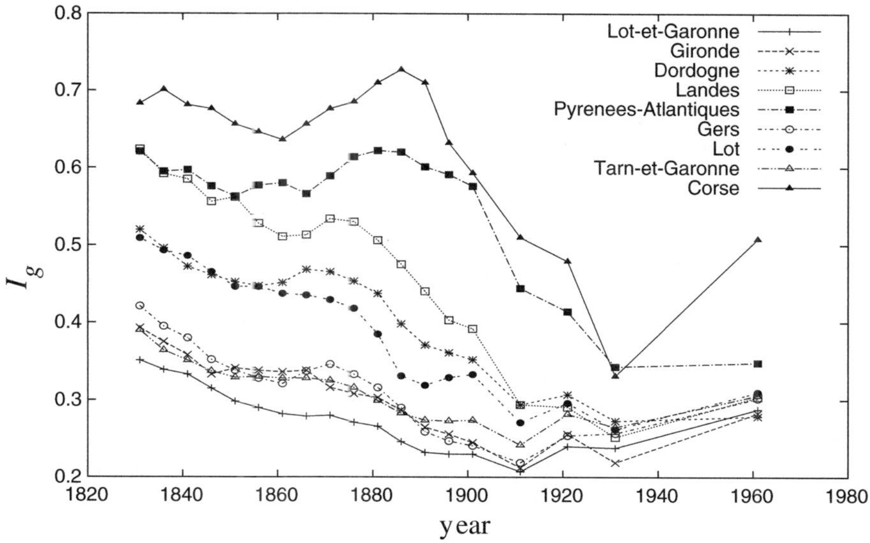

Fig. 2.20 The decline of I_g in Aquitaine and parts of Midi-Pyrénées. *Source* Ansley J. Coale and Roy Treadway [13]. The data shown in Table 2.6 are depicted here as a *line graph*

at other points should have reverted to the locus of the reaction-diffusion process. This occurrence suggests the potent and unvarying strength of the reaction-diffusion. While countermeasures against the falling birth rate may temporarily increase the mean number of children of each set of parents, their effects are soon exhausted in the reaction-diffusion process. It is impossible to expect such extensive and continuous economic development, which occurred during the nineteenth century, to be repeated in present day developed countries.

2.6 Districts Situated 600–500 km Away from the Singularity

It is essential to note that the onset date of fertility decline within a particular location in France, depended almost exclusively on its distance from the singularity. These phenomena provide us with decisive evidence of the background independence of fertility decline.

As I have already noted, the data of Coale and Treadway are from 1831. The singularity occurred in around 1770, so a period of 60 years had passed by 1831. The progressive wave had traveled a distance of approximately 600 km in this period. This meant that I_g should have monotonically declined in départments within a 600 km radius of Lot-et-Garonne, and that the decline of I_g should not be observed beyond that radius.

Bourgogne is located at a distance of about 500 km from Lot-et-Garonne. In this district, fertility decline resulting from a process of reaction-diffusion had started on time. I_g had declined in all of the départments, for example, Côte-d'Or, which is famous for its Bourgogne wine, Nièvie, Saône-et-Loire, and Yonne, which produces "Chablis", a reputed white wine.

J. Fourier was born in Auxerre in the Yonne département in 1768. As the progressive wave had not reached Yonne, it is not at all surprising that he was the nineteenth child of a tailor.

Aube (Aube), Haute-Marne, Haute-Saone, Doubs are all located at a distance of about 600 km from Lot-et-Garonne. We can confirm that I_g declined in each of these départments.

The location of Haute-Normandie region is at the furthest point within the range of access of the progressive wave.This wave had reached Eure, which is relatively close to the singularity in 1831. However, we cannot confirm whether it had already reached Seine-Maritime, which is further away from the singularity than Eure.

The progressive wave reached Finistère (Bretagne) in 1831. However fertility in this area was originally high, leading to the belief among the early diffusionists that fertility decline was delayed here compared with other French districts.

2.7 Districts Located Further than 600 km Away from the Singularity

The progressive wave did not reach the départments that were situated beyond a 600 km radius of Lot-et-Garonne.

Pas-de-Calais is located at a distance of 700 km from the singularity. Nord is near the border with Belgium. These areas had not yet encountered the progressive wave. We can observe fluctuations of I_g from 1831 up to the 1850s. Subsequently, their fertility increased as a result of the French industrial revolution.

I would like my readers to recall from chapter one that in 1890, Charles de Gaulle was born in Lille (Nord départment) as the third out of five children. Since the occurrence of the singularity in 1770, 120 years had passed. Lille is located at a distance of about 740 km from Lot-et-Garonne. Thus, the progressive wave reached Lille after 74 years. In 1890, Lille was still in the midst of the of reaction-diffusion process. Because of the effect of the French industrial revolution, fertility in Nord remained relatively high. Thus, de Gaulle's parents merely behaved in conformity with their neighbors.

2.7.1 Advanced Industrial Development in Nord-Pas-de-Calais

The region of Nord-Pas-de-Calais, which has favorable geographical conditions, was one of the relatively advanced industrialized areas in 1831. This region provided high quality steel ore and coal and was a port for relaying these items to England. With its favorable climate conditions, it was industrialized, like Lorraine, at an early stage of the French industrialization process.

The fact that fertility decline did not commence in this region in 1830, and that agricultural regions were the predecessors regarding fertility decline, suggests the fallacy of the industrialization hypothesis. Moreover, it indicates the background independence of fertility decline.

In 1831, the progressive wave had not reached the Lorraine region. It had not arrived in the Muse département located near the border with Belgium. The lack of data for Moselle, Bas-Rhine prevented me from making any observations for this area.

2.7.2 Low Fertility in Northern France

Fairly low fertility was indicated for Paris and its peripheral départments, for example, Oise, Somme, and Eure in the 1830s. In particular, Eure's I_g was lower than that of Lot-et-Garonne. However it is almost certain that a singularity did not occur in northern France, judging by the arrival date of the progressive wave. In 1861, during the reign of Napoleon III, I_g increased again.[11] Thus, a singularity evidently did not occur in northern France.

The map included at the end of *The Decline of Fertility in Europe* (Fig. 1.4) indicates low I_g in 1870 in Paris and its peripheral areas, and in departments situated in areas along the national border. However, the low fertility in these areas can be attributed first to the high infant mortality caused by the custom of no breast feeding second to the riots and disturbances caused by the French Revolution, by Napoleon I, the July Revolution, and the French Revolution of 1848.

2.7.3 The Reaction-Diffusion Process in Belgium

It is apparent that fertility decline in Belgium was caused by the reaction-diffusion process. We can provide a fairly good description of the phases of fertility decline for each of the cities in Belgium from 1880 to 1900, based on the reaction-diffusion process.

[11] See Fig. 2.20 and Table 2.6. I_g did not increase in the Lot-et-Garonne singularity. The singularity had maintained the lowest marital fertility during the process of reaction-diffusion.

Table 2.7 Decline of I_g for provinces in Belgium

	Mons	Chalerol	Dinant	Namur	Bruxelles	Liege	Arlon
1880	0.526	0.596	0.663	0.646	0.673	0.688	0.730
1890	0.472	0.478	0.573	0.571	0.570	0.577	0.650
1900	0.382	0.390	0.511	0.485	0.470	0.470	0.582
	Antwerpen	Leuven	Bastogne	Hasselt	Kortrijk	Ostende	
1880	0.810	0.849	0.854	0.868	0.894	0.899	
1890	0.713	0.806	0.804	0.818	0.853	0.905	
1900	0.584	0.751	0.756	0.865	0.812	0.800	

Source Ansley J. Coale and Roy Treadway [13]. Data after 1910 are omitted

Suppose that the progressive wave traveled from the direction of Lot-et-Garonne in southwestern France. This assumption leads to the belief that fertility decline was delayed in the northwestern provinces of Belgium.

We can definitely verify this belief (see Table 2.7 and Fig. 2.21. In the national border areas between France and Belgium, the southern areas experienced fertility decline earlier than the northern areas. Mons, which is at a distance of 740 km from Lot-et-Garonne demonstrated a decline of I_g earlier than Kortrijk, which is at a distance of 760 km from Lot-et-Garonne. Fertility decline in northern Belgian cities such as Ostende, Antwerpen, and Hasselt was delayed compared with southern cities.

Although Bruxelles, located in central Belgium, is the national capital and an industrial, economic, and political center, fertility decline in this city was delayed compared with that of southern Mons, Chalerol, and Namur. This fact is further evidence of the background independence of fertility decline.

Readers may perceive the relatively late decline of I_g in southeastern Belgium, namely, Arlon and Bastogne to be an inconsistency. One of the properties of a progressive wave is that it stagnates in highlands and plateaus where the population is sparse. Consequently, it slowed down in Ardennes. This accounted for the delay of fertility decline in southeastern Belgium.

The following figure depicts the declining I_g of each Belgian city. Figure 2.20 on p. 63 resembles Fig. 2.22. The question, then, is why did the fertility decline process in southwestern France (Aquitaine) that occurred 60 years earlier in what was still an agricultural area resemble that which occurred in Belgium, where industry was considerably developed? This coincidence suggests that an identical reaction-diffusion process occurred in both areas. It implies that the reaction-diffusion process proceeds in a way that does not depend on the socioeconomic background.

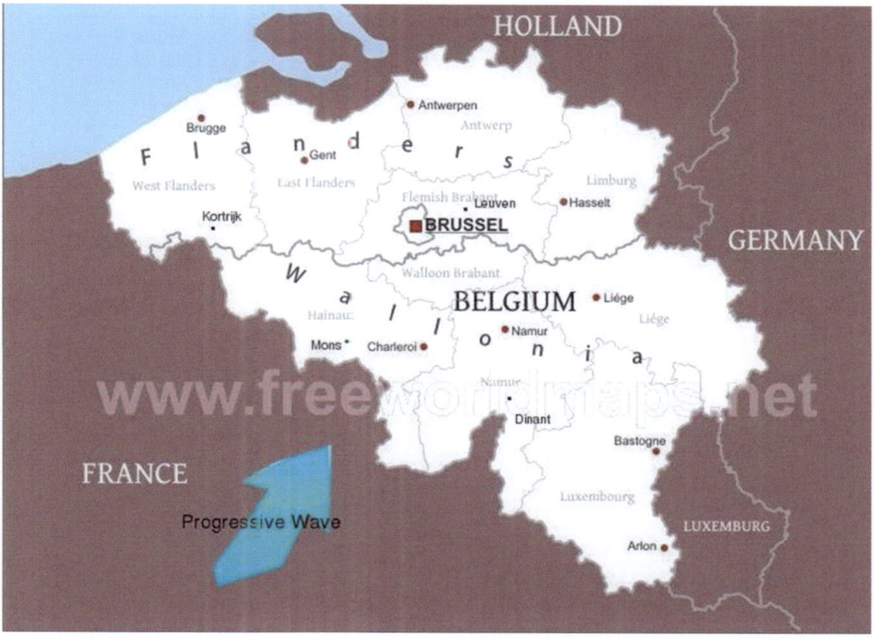

Fig. 2.21 Map of Belgium. *Source* http://www.freeworldmaps.net/europe/belgium/political.html. I have added some cities to the map, as well as an *arrow* indicating the direction of the progressive wave

2.7.3.1 The Solution of Industrial and Cultural Differences in Fertility Decline in Belgium

To examine fertility decline of Belgium from the perspective of a reaction-diffusion process may also enable us to solve a question that remains unsettled. This refers to the contradiction relating to the industrialization hypothesis that was raised by the initial diffusionists.

I will request my readers to return to Table 1.1 on p. 3. This indicates from the "Date of Decline in Marital Fertility by 10 %" that fertility decline occurred earlier in Belgium (1882) than in the Netherlands (1897). However other socioeconomic indices such as infant mortality and percentages of rural areas and cities with populations over 20,000 indicate greater advancement of the Netherlands compared with Belgium, at least in terms of industrialization. If the industrialization hypothesis is true, then fertility decline in both countries occurred out of sequence.

The conception that the progressive wave of fertility decline had been diffusing from Lot-et-Garonne solves this contradiction. The progressive wave must have passed Belgium to reach the Netherlands in the reverse direction to that followed by advancing German armies during both WWI and WWII. It took ten years for the progressive wave to reach the Netherlands from the France-Belgium border, because it was traveling at a velocity of 10 km/year. This solution to the contradiction is further evidence of background independence.

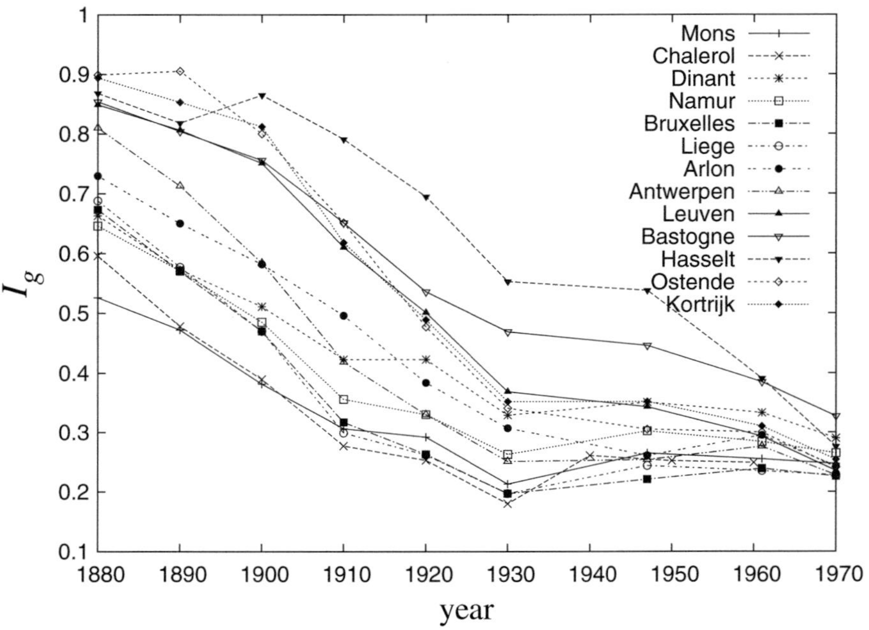

Fig. 2.22 Decline of I_g in each city in Belgium

This simple explanation provided by the reaction-diffusion hypothesis can solve another question concerning Belgium's fertility decline. The early diffusionists believed that cultural differences between the Flemish and Walloon communities caused the difference in the tempo of fertility decline. The hypothesis that the linguistic difference between the Flemish community within a Dutch-speaking area and the Walloon community within a French-speaking area was the underlying factor causing the difference in the tempo of fertility decline was widely accepted.

In fact, this language distribution perfectly matches the geographical distribution of Belgium's population (please refer again to Figs. 2.21 and 2.23. The progressive wave first touched the southern portion of Belgium, which is a French-speaking

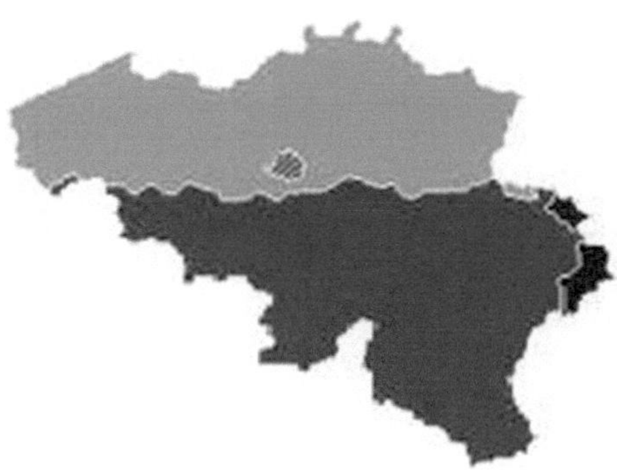

Fig. 2.23 Belgian communities. The North is a Dutch-speaking area inhabited by the Flemish community; the South is a French-speaking area inhabited by the Walloon community, and the East is inhabited by the German-speaking community. *Source* http://en.wikipedia.org/wiki/Belgium

area and the home of the Walloon community. It did not reach the Flemish community/Dutch-speaking area until it had passed through the Walloon community. Thus, the geographical distribution of the linguistic population and the advancing route taken by the progressive wave did result in a cultural difference relating to fertility decline.

However, if we had instead divided Belgium into western and eastern communities, we would not have observed any differences in fertility decline related to community and language. Thus, the reaction-diffusion process is also independent of the cultural background. The background naturally entails cultural factors.

2.8 Conclusion

To postulate a reaction-diffusion process for fertility decline in Europe, Japan, and other countries results in novel findings. Accordingly, we can estimate the velocity of diffusion and discover the origin (singularity) of fertility decline. Consequently, I estimate that fertility decline originated in *Lot-et Garonne* around 1770.

By applying the reaction-diffusion model, we can explain the fertility decline process in Europe, both longitudinally and geographically. Even though we cannot exclude the possibility that socioeconomic conditions played an important role in the occurrence of singularity, they actually played a minor role in the middle of this process. Rapid economic growth during the reign of Napoleon III did indeed lead to a temporary increase in French fertility from the 1860s to 1870s. However, at the conclusion of this period of economic growth, French fertility declined again, as has been captured by the trajectory of decline. Fertility decline caused by Reaction-diffusion was independent of its background.

Chapter 3
Marriage Function as an Integral Equation

Abstract If we agree that fertility decline occurs independently of background, we can further assume that marriages occur independently of their background. Moreover, we can express a theoretical marriage function that is background-independent as an integral equation. We begin by critically examining existing marriage functions, namely, the Coale-McNeil distribution, double exponential distribution, and the Hernes' function. Guided by critical analyses of Hernes' differential equation, I propose an integral equation as a marriage function based on a simple marriage model. This assumes that the probability of first marriage occurrence completely depends on the ratio of women in their first marriage within a given space. This also implies background independence of the marriage function. This integral equation not only fits the observed data well, but also provides the most likely estimations of the mean age at first marriage. This is decisive evidence that my proposed integral equation is the most reliable marriage function. To formulate marriage function is one of the requirements for predicting fertility.

Keywords Marriage function · Coale-McNeil Distribution · Hernes function · Integral equation · Background independence

3.1 Introduction to Marriage Function

We can observe a unique distribution pattern for age at first marriage, as shown in Fig. 3.3. This unique pattern leads us to the conception that there is an unknown fundamental law that governs these phenomena. Starting with "Coale-McNeil distribution", we began our search for the function demonstrating the best fit. However, in addition to a good fit, it must also entail a reasonable behavioral model for deducing marriage function.

Thus, we need a model of first marriage occurrences. Viewing marriage as a stochastic event that occurs within a given and limited space-time point, it is relatively easy for us to construct a simple model of first marriages. We are unable to accurately determine when we will get married over our long life spans. In this chapter, I adopt the stochastic behavioral paradigm, which posits that the occurrence of first marriage

S. Ike, *Fertility Decline and Background Independence*,
Population Studies of Japan, DOI 10.1007/978-4-431-55151-5_3

is random at the macro scale. The perception that we ourselves subjectively decide whether or not to get married is a trivial concern within a theory of marriage function.

When we express first marriages occurrences as a computable equation, we can predict these occurrences numerically. Thus the theory that I introduce in this chapter allows for falsifiability.

Marriage is the first necessary event in fertility behavior. Obtaining the probability density function of marriage occurrences is thus the first indispensable step for studying fertility.

3.2 Previous Marriage Functions

3.2.1 Coale-McNeil Distribution: A Convolution Model

In 1971, Coale found that the distribution pattern of age at first marriage was unique [11]. Based on his analysis of data from Sweden, he empirically proposed double exponential distribution.

$$p(t) = 0.174 \exp(-4.411 \exp(-0.309\, t)) \tag{3.1}$$

The following year, in collaboration with McNeil, he proposed the Coale-McNeil [9] distribution model (Eq. (3.2)). This is a convolution of a quasi-normal distribution and three exponential distributions. The quasi-normal distribution corresponds to physiological maturity. The latter three distributions correspond to being acquainted, engaged, and married, respectively.

$$F(t) = \frac{\lambda}{\Gamma(\alpha/\lambda)} \exp(-\alpha(t-\mu) - \exp(-\lambda(t-\mu))) \tag{3.2}$$

The Coale-McNeil distribution does appear to bear a relation to the actual marriage process. However, when we consider common-law marriages that have prevailed over a long period of time, then the marriage process that is assumed within the Coale-McNeil distribution is inaccurate. Legal marriage procedures are not the same as the occurrence of marriage itself.

Moreover, although less parsimonious, the fit of the Coale-McNeil distribution is no better than the fit of other double exponential distributions. The Coale-McNeil distribution has three parameters, which is more than those of general double exponential distributions. In addition, the Coale-McNeil distribution shares a crucial defect in that the integration of $F(t)$ easily converges to one as with other double exponential distributions.

3.2.2 Applications of Extreme Events

The Coale-McNeil distribution is a variation of of double exponential distribution in its expression. Double exponential distributions (Eq. (3.3), Fig. 3.1) are usually applied to the life of manufactured products or the time between failures. First marriage occurrences within a cohort resemble the failures of products manufactured during the same period.

$$f(t) = a\exp(-a(t-\mu) - \exp(-a(t-\mu))) \tag{3.3}$$

Normally the weakest part of a product causes its failure. That is to say, just one failure can cause the failure of the whole product. **This leads us to the consequential inference that first marriages occur as one critical event and not as the sufficiency of several conditions.** This appears incredible to our subjective consciousness. This suggestive implication has long escaped our notice. If double exponential distributions are good approximations of the function of first marriage, we should accept the inference that they only occur as one stochastic event. Convolution models such as the Coale-McNeil distribution assume the sufficiency of four conditions. We have now seen that convolution models essentially conflict with double exponential distributions, with the exception of the convolution of infinite random variables. The Coale-McNeil distribution is a convolution of four random variables. Consequently, it differs fundamentally from double exponential distributions.

Undoubtedly, double exponential distributions are no more than exclusive approximations of the function of first marriage, because we cannot interpret alterations of

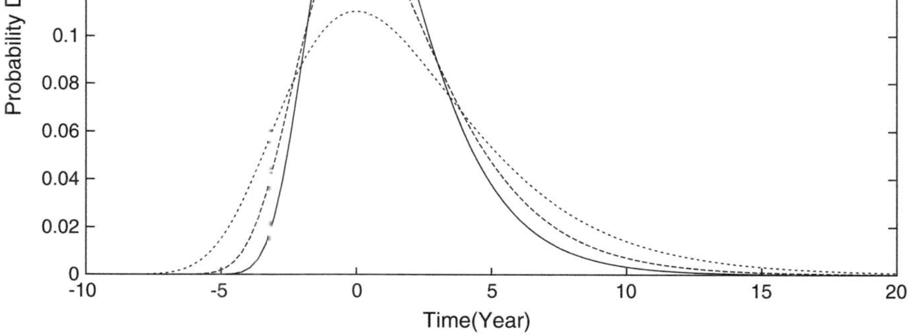

Fig. 3.1 Double exponential distributions

its coefficients in the contexts of real societies. Double exponential distributions (including that of Coale-McNeil) have a critical defect, which is that their integration converges rapidly to one. Empirical data have suggested that marriage functions must not have such a property within human society. Accordingly, Coale and his supporters first empirically excluded the never married population (for example, 5 %) from their denominator of a cohort before recalculating the probabilities of first marriages. The true function of first marriages must entail non-empirical (namely theoretical) prediction of the ratio of never married individuals within a cohort in any given period. Accordingly, double exponential distributions are questionable marriage functions.

In Fig. 3.3, this defect of the double exponential function is evident in the shapes of the distributions. The observed data have relative higher skewness than double exponential distribution, especially in the half of their distribution on the left side. When we make a fit to the observed data in accordance with its mode, after the mode, the double exponential and the Coale-McNeil distributions have evident relative thicker probability densities than the observed data.

3.3 How First Marriages Occur

From my previous considerations, I have deduced that marriage occurs as one random event and not as a synthesis of several events. If this is the case, then how does such a random event occur? My answer to this question is that its occurrence depends on neighboring occurrences of marriage. G. Hernes [29] proposed a very correlative model in relation to this view.

3.3.1 Hernes' Function

Hernes constructed a model of entry into marriage using a differential equation.

$$\frac{dP_t}{dt} = Ab^t(1 - P_t)P_t \tag{3.4}$$

P_t is the ratio of the first-time married population within a cohort. We should keep in mind the basic relation between the ratio of the first-time married population and the probability density of first marriage. Namely, the derivative of the ratio of the first-time married population is the probability density of first marriage. Let $F(t)$ be the probability density of first marriage at time t. We can express the following equation:

$$\frac{dP_t}{dt} = F(t) = Ab^t(1 - P_t)P_t \tag{3.5}$$

Consequently the probability density of first marriage varies, depending on P_t and $(1 - P_t)$. Hernes' function assumes that marriage occurrences depend only on neighboring marriage occurrences except for the effect of b^t.

3.3.2 Flaws of Hernes' Function

I assume that Hernes was obliged to introduce coefficients A and b^t to fit the equation to the observed data. He defined these coefficients as follows: A is the average initial marriageability and $b < 1$ its constant of deterioration.

An equation that explains a phenomenon has to have at least one coefficient. Setting aside coefficient A, for the fit with the observed data, the marriage function must have a monotonic decreasing element. Consequently, Hernes adopted the exponential function b^t. However, in my opinion, these definitions and interpretations of parameters are unreasonable.

3.3.3 The More Marriages That are Evident Within a Space, the Higher the Occurrences of Marriage

We are strongly inclined to get married when there are many marriages occurring within our cohort in a given space. Thus, marriage probability $F(t)$ is proportional to $\int_0^t F(t)(dt)$. In contrast to this tendency, when there are fewer unmarried persons within our cohort, the probability of being selected for marriage is reduced. We initially express $F(t)$ as the following equation:

$$F(t) = \lambda \int_0^t F(t)(dt) \left(1 - \int_0^t F(t)(dt)\right) \left(\text{unknown element}\right) \tag{3.6}$$

This integral equation corresponds to Hernes' each elements $AP_t(1 - P_t)$. However, we require a substitute for b^t that decreases monotonically in the space in which marriages occur.

3.3.3.1 A Monotonic Decreasing Element

The most important considerations for marriage functions are whether the monotonic decreasing element is appropriate for the fit and whether it provides a reasonable explanation of the phenomena. In this regard, the right tail of the distribution of marriage functions is the decisive discriminant test to judge the correctness of existing marriage functions.

We can readily observe that the distribution of first marriages has a long, thick, and respectable right tail (see Figs. 3.3, 3.4). This implies that people continue to enter into first marriages at relatively older ages (35–50, and even over 60 years). Empirical data suggest a correlation between fewer marriage occurrences at younger ages and more occurrences at older ages. Therefore, the rapid decrement of the exponential function of t is a lethal attribute for marriage function. Considering this from another angle, a monotonic decreasing element in a true marriage function has the characteristic of fewer marriages occurring at younger ages and more marriages occurring at older ages. However, Hernes' b^t lacks this important property. The monotonic decreasing element in marriage function must be a variable that is dependent on the tempo of marriage occurrences.

3.3.3.2 Monotonic Decrease in the Never Married Ratio

The probability of first marriage occurrences depend on the ratio of those who have never married at time t. This ratio shows a monotonic decrease with t. The monotonic decreasing element to be included in an equation of first marriage function must be the ratio of those who have never married.

3.3.4 Formulation of an Integral Equation

Strictly considering the continuity of time as a real number, $\dfrac{dP}{dt}$ is zero almost everywhere, because marriage does not occur within an arbitrary and very short interval. Therefore, marriage occurrences must be expressed as a Lebesgue integration.[1]

The ratio of the category "ever married" is the sum of the probability of the occurrence of marriage. Thus, $P(t) = \int_0^t F(t)(dt)$. We, therefore, obtain the following integral equation for the probability of marriage $F(t)$ at time t.

$$F(t) = \lambda \int_0^t F(t)(dt) \left(1 - \int_0^t F(t)(dt)\right) \left(1 - \int_0^t F(t)(dt)\right) \tag{3.7}$$

$F(t)$ is defined within a measurable space. Consequently, F (*first marriage occurrences) belongs entirely to an additive class. Henceforth, we will refer to this integral equation as a Space Dependent Stochastic Marriage Function (3.7) **SDSMF**, because $F(t)$ varies depending on the ratio of the ever married within its space.

---

[1] "(dt)" indicates that this integration is a Lebesgue integration. The Riemann-Stielties integration is expressed as $\int F(t)dt$.

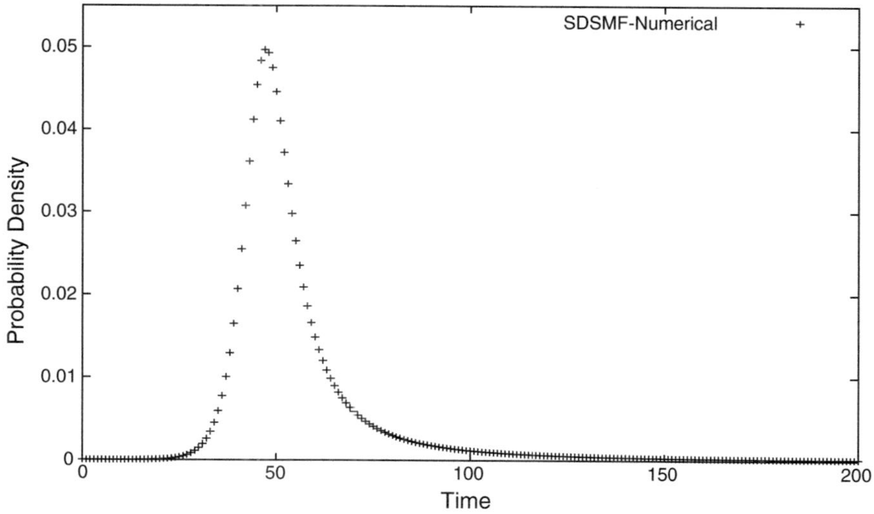

Fig. 3.2 Numeric solution of SDSMF

3.3.4.1 Characteristics of SDSMF—Thicker Right Tail and Higher Kurtosis

We cannot solve the integral equation (3.7) analytically. However, we can easily solve it numerically (see Fig. 3.2).

We can readily observe that SDSMF has a thicker right tail than that of the double exponential distribution. Consequently kurtosis is higher than for the Coale-McNeil or double exponential distributions (*see Fig. 3.3). Observed frequencies of first marriages express this relative higher kurtosis.

3.3.4.2 Background Independence of Marriage Occurrences

It is important that the integral equation (3.7) is only dependent on the integration of $F(t)$ of t. Thus, the ratio of first marriages develops by itself, independently from other socioeconomic conditions. I refer to this property as background independence of marriage occurrences. Though we have entertained a vague belief that socioeconomic conditions affect marriage occurrences, people themselves decide this stochastically and independently of prevailing socioeconomic conditions. Marriages occur atomically and are dependent on their own quantum in just the same way as other animal manner.

Consequently, we are able to infer that the distribution of first marriages is decided by means of itself in the present. We can foresee the consequences and conclusions of the first marriages of each cohort when we examine the initial occurrences of first

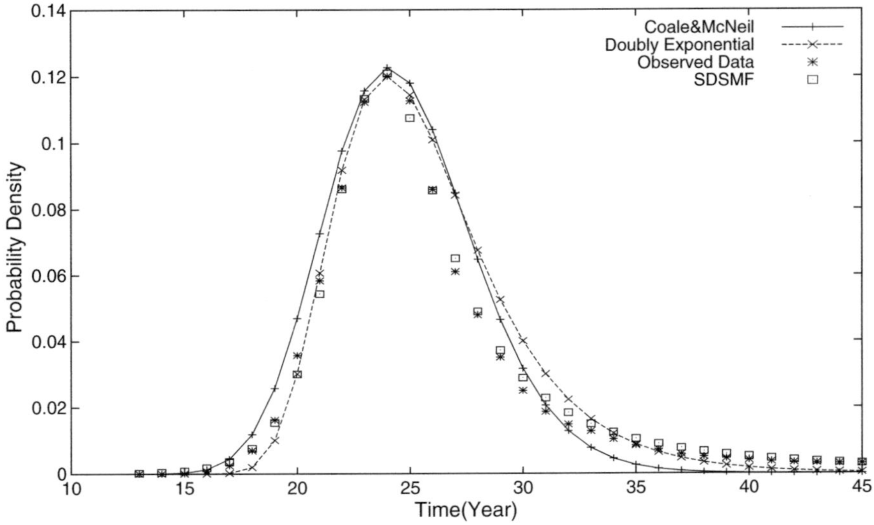

Fig. 3.3 Coale-McNeil and doubly exponential distributions for the observed 1960 Japanese cohort and SDSMF adjusted at the inflection point

marriage for each cohort. An exception, however, is the extraordinary and large-scale historical event known as the "Baby Boom."[2]

3.3.5 The Fit of SDSMF with the Data

To fit SDSMF with the observed data, we require the concrete values of the coefficients λ and the interval of time t corresponding to the actual time (year). The time interval of SDSMF is supposed to be much shorter than a year. Therefore the appropriate values of the time interval of SDSMF are integrated (summed up) to achieve a fit with the probability of first marriage observed by year.

3.3.5.1 The Inflection Point Method

To estimate parameter λ and interval t, I freshly developed the inflection point method. This finds the most likely λ by means of the correspondence of SDSMF's inflection point to the observed inflection point.

The ratio of first-time married individuals of a cohort at a specific age (an endpoint) is not sufficient for estimating parameters. The observed ratio of individuals who have

[2]However, even the "Baby Boom" is not an exception for SDSMF. Its onset occurred as a mere historical accident, and its subsequent durability can be explained by SDSMF.

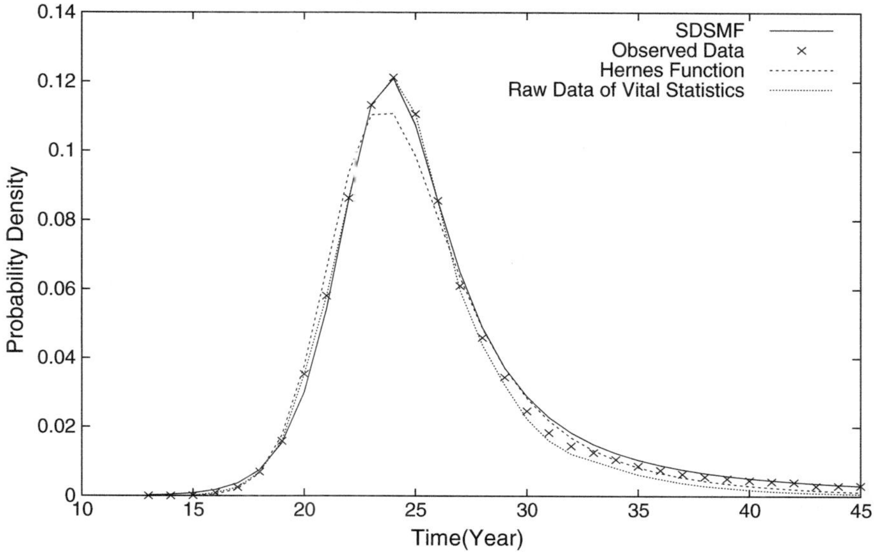

Fig. 3.4 SDSMF and Hernes' function for the 1960 Japanese cohort and observed data

ever been married, aged 45 or 50 years, is far from the true values, because there are too many common-law marriages within older age groups that are not declared publicly. I do not consider the endpoint of the marriage process to be suitable for estimating marriage features. However, in contrast to the imprecision of the endpoint, the inflection point is relatively accurate.

3.3.5.2 The Results of Estimation

I adopted SDSMF for the first marriages of several Japanese cohorts, applying the inflection point method. There was a good fit (average absolute error < 0.00159427 for each age) with the observed values[3] of first marriages for the 1960 Japanese cohort. The fit was, however, best for the 1950 Japanese cohort. The inflection method accomplished an average absolute error < 0.000932. It missed less than 0.1 %, on average, for annual observations.

The inflection method estimates λ at $\simeq .22$. I have assumed that λ is a constant and interval t alters because the dependency on the neighboring ratio of ever married individuals is universal. The tempo of neighboring first marriage occurrences thus alters the macro tempo of first marriage occurrences.

[3]Observed values were calculated from vital statistics that were modified in accordance with the census.

3.4 Decisive Evidence of SDSMF

A good fit is not in itself a strong test of the validity of the marriage function as described by Hernes below.

> The general problem with our type of analysis is that the fit between the observed and calculated curve of first marriages in itself is not a strong test of the model. Since the model is the only link between the data and the assumed substantive casual processes (measured by the parameters), it is hard to tell whether the resulting estimates actually reflect the casual forces involved.
>
> Hernes [29], p.180

So he brought attention to the necessities of the demonstrative test as following.

> A much stronger test of the causal forces represented by the parameters would be to derive alternative measures of them, or to confront other empirical consequences of the model with data.
>
> Hernes [29], p.181

Thus, Hernes drew attention to the necessity of a demonstrative test.

I propose a corroborative and novel test for marriage functions, described below, that merits the "scientific" label.

3.4.1 A Good Theory Can Predict Some Theoretical Values

The critical issue is whether a theory can enable the prediction of real and theoretical values. With SDSMF, we can predict the average age at first marriage for a cohort as an expected value. It is then easy to calculate the mean age of the first-time married population with SDSMF, because SDSMF is a probability density function.

We can certainly calculate the average age at first marriage for a cohort from vital statistics. However, this age is always lower than the true value. The reason for this is that people tend not to declare their marriages when they marry at older ages. Thus, we cannot know the true value of the average age at first marriage from vital statistics.

$$\text{Mean Age at first marriage} = \int_0^t t\ F(t)(dt) \tag{3.8}$$

The formula for the calculation is as follows:

$$\text{Mean Age at first marriage} = \sum_0^t t\ F(t_i) \tag{3.9}$$

From the estimated values of $F(t)$, I calculated the theoretical expected mean age at first marriage (see Table 3.1). I then compared this to the observed value, the

Table 3.1 Theoretical mean age at first marriage for the 1960 Japanese cohort

Age at	SDSMF prediction	Observed from vital statistics	Hernes function prediction
45	24.329481	23.410084	23.033714

Table 3.2 Average ages at first marriage from data samples of the 1960 cohort calculated from social surveys

Survey	Year	$\overline{x}$	n	s
JGSS	2000–2002	24.8219	73	3.42119
NFR, JGSS	1998, 2000–2, 2006	24.7883212	137	3.5405854

calculated value according to the Hernes' function, and the estimations from the Japanese General Social Survey (JGSS) samples. Each of these values is exhibited in Table 3.2.

When we assume a somewhat higher standard deviation $\sigma = 3.6$, we estimate the 95 % confidence interval as [23.996, 25.648]. Only SDSMF's prediction falls within this range, though it is still smaller than the estimation calculated for the Japanese General Social Survey (JGSS) samples. I suggest that SDSMF's prediction is the most probable.

Let us examine this problem as a statistical test. It is a landmark outcome for the social sciences that we are able to frame an alternative point hypothesis and a null point hypothesis not as a trivial zero.

$$\begin{cases} H_0 : \mu = 24.329481 \\ H_1 : \mu = 23.410084 \end{cases} \tag{3.10}$$

Normally within the social sciences, we can only test a null hypothesis as $\mu = 0,\ \beta = 0$. The null hypothesis is only used for falsification. This test is identically lenient for the alternative hypothesis, $\mu \neq 0,\ \beta \neq 0$, which is verified against the null hypothesis. It is almost always true that $\mu\, and\ \beta$ are not equal to zero within populations for several reasons.

As long as we cannot hypothesize a concrete null point hypothesis and a point alternative hypothesis that have the ring of truth, the null hypothesis can always be rejected by applying the statistical test,[4] especially when we can make calculations for as many samples as we want. We are not able to determine the power of previous statistical tests within the social sciences.

In contrast to this lenient test, I hypothesize H_0 for the verification from a more rigorous standpoint. Even when confined to this statistical test problem, SDSMF is demonstrably more sufficient than other existing marriage theories. No other theories are able to theoretically predict the true mean age at first marriage.

[4]This is an incorrect tradition that originated with L.R. Klein. We must abandon this improper way of conducting a statistical test in favor of a theory that is able to hypothesize a point null hypothesis that is not trivial.

Table 3.3 Calculated ratios of the ever married populations of the cohort for each function and estimations

SDSMF	Observed	Coale-McNeil	Doubly exp	JGSS	n
0.93929	0.91332	0.997039	0.99670	0.94118	119
		-		0.93483	445
*information, Census 2000 for Age 40–44, 45–49				0.91418	0.91795

3.4.1.1 The Result of a Test

I selected samples from the 1960 cohort from JGSS 2000–2002, JGSS, 2006, and NFRJ, 1998.[5] I then calculated estimations for average age and an associated standard deviation for the 1960 cohort in Japan as follows: $\overline{x} = 24.7883212, s = 3.5405854, n = 137$. If we assume that $\sigma = 3.6$, which is somewhat higher than the expected, the critical regions of H_0 are $[-\infty, 23.727]\, and\ [24.932, \infty]$ for a 0.05 level of significance. We accept H_0.

We can then calculate the probability of error of the second kind β and, consequently, the power of the test.

$$\frac{23.727 - 23.4100842}{3.6}\sqrt{137} \doteq 0.98 \Rightarrow P\{z > 0.98\} \doteq 0.16354 \qquad (3.11)$$

$\beta \doteq 0.16354$. The power of this test is $0.83 <$. Accordingly, H_0 is more likely to be true. That is to say, SDSMF is a valid function that describes the actual process of first marriage. It is a theoretical triumph of SDSMF that it is able to precisely predict the average age at first marriage of the 1960 cohort in Japan.

3.4.2 Comparing SDSMF to the Coale-McNeil and Double Exponential Distributions

3.4.2.1 The Decisive Discriminant Test

A critical difference of SDSMF compared with the Coale-McNeil distribution is that it does not easily converge to zero. It also takes a considerably longer time than double exponential distributions to integrate SDSMF to 1. This property of SDSMF implies that it includes the never married population of a cohort within the equation itself. SDSMF is able to predict the ratio of the never married population at time t. We can calculate the expected ratio of the population that is ever married within a cohort at time t soon after the marriage process begins (from ages 16 or 17 years). I present the expected ratios for each marriage function in Table 3.3.

[5]National Family Research of Japan 1998 was conducted by the Japan Society of Family Sociology.

3.4.2.2 The Ratio of the Ever Married Population for the 1960 Cohort

Let us perform a simple statistical test for the ratio of the ever married population within the 1960 Japanese cohort. Let p be the ratio of the ever married population aged 45 years. For the 2000–2003 JGSS sample, for which $n = 119$, we obtained the estimation of $\hat{p} = 1 - 0.05882 = 0.94118$. Assuming $\sigma^2 \doteq 0.9 \times 0.1 = 0.09$ to be somewhat larger than the parameter of the population, we calculated a 95 % confidence interval for p [0.88728, 0.99508]. The original plain (not adjusted in accordance with the census) data of vital statistics, and the Coale-McNeil, and double exponential distributions are excluded.

There are too few samples to be able to perform a one proportion z-test for $n = 119$. I combined the following samples: JGSS2006, NFRJ98, NFRJ01, NFRJ03, and SSM1995.[6] Consequently, I acquired $n = 445$ samples for the 1960 Japanese cohort. I obtained the 95 % confidence interval as [0.90696, 0.96270]. SDSMF and the observed values were included.

Let us now perform the one proportion z-test.

$$\begin{cases} H_0 : p = 0.93929 \\ H_1 : p = 0.99670 \end{cases} \tag{3.12}$$

Assuming a somewhat large $\sigma^2 \doteq 0.09$, and setting the level of significance at 0.05, we obtain the following region of rejection: [0, 0.91142] and [0.96716, 1]. The value $\hat{p} = 0.93483$ does not reject H_0. The power of the test is 0.984. Thus, we can exclude double exponential and Coale-McNeil distributions from the group of reasonable marriage functions with considerable certainty.

This demonstrates the power of the property of background independence and of the integral equation of SDSMF. SDSMF is a natural expression of a marriage process and enables us to calculate the ratio of the unmarried population at time t.

3.5 Testing SDSMF in Other Countries

It is necessary to test the validity of SDSMF for other countries. I posit that the integral equation describes a universal process of first marriage occurrences. Thus, background independence of marriage occurrences is worth examining for several additional countries.

By conducting these test procedures, I was able to determine whether or not the theory could predict the rate of early marriage occurrences, which is also a decisive feature of marriage function.

---

[6]Japanese Social Stratification and Mobility Survey, 1995.

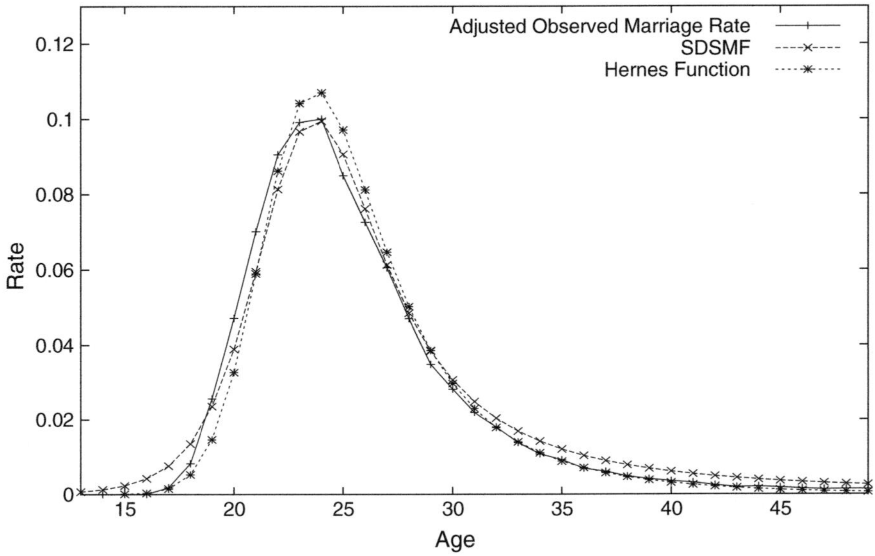

Fig. 3.5 Observed first marriage rate and SDSMF for the 1924 Swiss cohort. *Source* G. Calot [5]

3.5.1 Testing SDSMF Using Cohorts Within the Swiss Population

3.5.1.1 Similarities to the Japanese Cases

Figures 3.5 and 3.6 shows the result of adaptation of SDSMF and Hernes' function to the first marriage rates of the 1924 and 1930 Swiss cohort.[7] We can clearly distinguish tendencies of each function that are similar to those we observed for Japan.

SDSMF estimates showed a higher marriage rate for older ages than what was observed. Hernes' function exhibited a good fit for both tails. However, in contrast to the tails, the fit was not good at the top.

For the right tail, we find that SDSMF is more reasonable than what we observed for Japan. There are good grounds for believing that more first marriages occur after the age of 35 years as common-law marriages. These are not even specified in the census questionnaire. I performed the same test for the 1940 Swiss cohort as for the Japanese cohort using ESS data.[8]

[7] I used data from *Two centuries of Swiss demographic history —Graphic album of the 1860–2050 period* [5].

[8] The European Social Survey (ESS) is an academically-driven social survey designed to chart and explain the interaction between Europe's changing institutions and the attitudes, beliefs and behavior patterns of its diverse populations. The ESS was established in 2001, and was led by its founder and coordinator, Roger Jowell, until his death in December 2011 (http://www.europeansocialsurvey.org/).

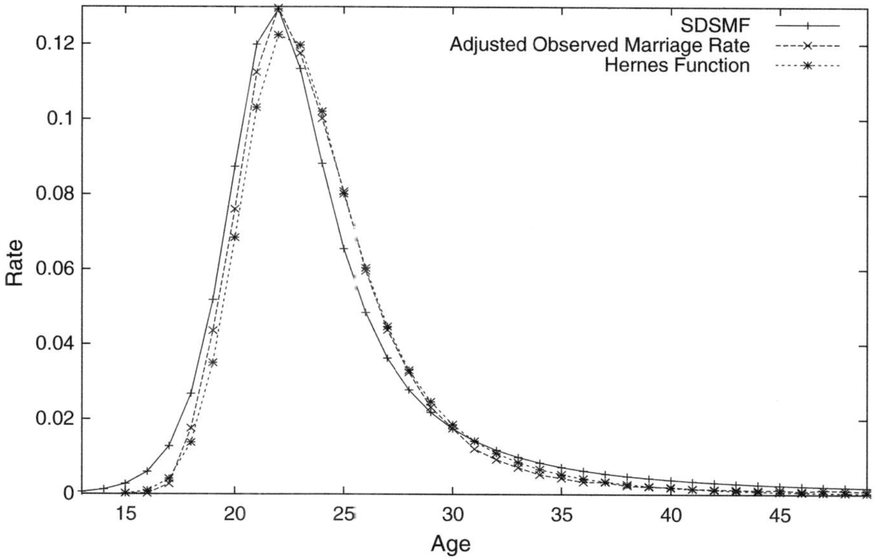

Fig. 3.6 Observed first marriage rate and SDSMF for the 1930 Swiss cohort. *Source* G. Calot [5]

$$\begin{cases} H_0 : p = 0.951243 \\ H_1 : p = 0.918378 \end{cases} \tag{3.13}$$

The region of rejection is $[0, 0.903031]$, $[1.0, 1.0]$. $\hat{p} = 0.939394$ does not reject H_0. Granted that the power of the test is poor, SDSMF's ratio is the most likely.

3.5.2 Marriage at Young Ages: The Second Decisive Discriminant Test

SDSMF systematically predicts that more marriages at young ages would occur compared with adjusted observed data or estimates using the Hernes' function. The question, then, is which of these is correct? Whether or not a theory can predict real rates of marriage occurrences at young ages is a definitive touchstone for the function of first marriages.

3.5.2.1 How Often Do Marriages at Young Ages Occur?

The Swiss federal statistical office does not record the marriages of individuals below the age of 15 years. However, the fact that there are no such records does not mean that marriages of individuals below 15 years do not occur.

Table 3.4 Age at first marriage in the US derived from General Social Survey (GSS) samples (http://www3.norc.org/GSS+Website/)

Age	Freq	Prob	Prob (vaild)
12	4	0.00013	0.00026
13	37	0.00125	0.00240
14	103	0.00347	0.00668
15	263	0.00886	0.01706
16	783	0.02639	0.05079
17	1247	0.04202	0.08090
⋮	⋮		
Total	14260	/26675	

Moreover, I think that the rate of occurrence of recorded marriage of individuals aged 16–18 years does not reflect real marriages, including cohabitant unions or common-law marriages, because they are too few in number. We should consider the physiological maturity of Caucasoids,[9] as more than a few probably developed cohabitant unions.

I extracted ages at first marriage from cumulative GSS[10] samples from the US. Table 3.4 presents the frequencies of occurrence of young marriages for the total cumulative samples.

SDSMF is an integral equation. If we accept the validity of SDSMF in relation to first marriage occurrences, they absolutely depend on the initial first marriage occurrences. This can be logically deduced from the background independence of marriage. The question of whether or not there are more marriages than registrations is decisively important.

In actual processes of marriage occurrences, neighboring occurrences of early marriages determine subsequent marriage occurrences within this cohort. So I have reflected on this consequence of the second decisive discriminant test, and consider that the occurrence of more marriages than those that are registered is much more probable. Nonetheless, a social survey that is meticulously designed to count early young marriages will resolve this problem.

3.5.3 A Test Using Algeria Data

L.Henry [28] recorded the marriage distribution of Muslims in Algeria in 1948. Let us apply SDSMF and the Hernes' function to this data (*see Fig. 3.7) SDSMF and the inflection point method are able to describe the distribution peak quite well. This presents an intriguing contrast in that the Hernes' function did not demonstrate a

[9]The concept of race is not scientific. Nonetheless I use "Caucasoid" to denote ethnic groups such as Anglo Saxons and Germans.

[10]http://www3.norc.org/gss+website/

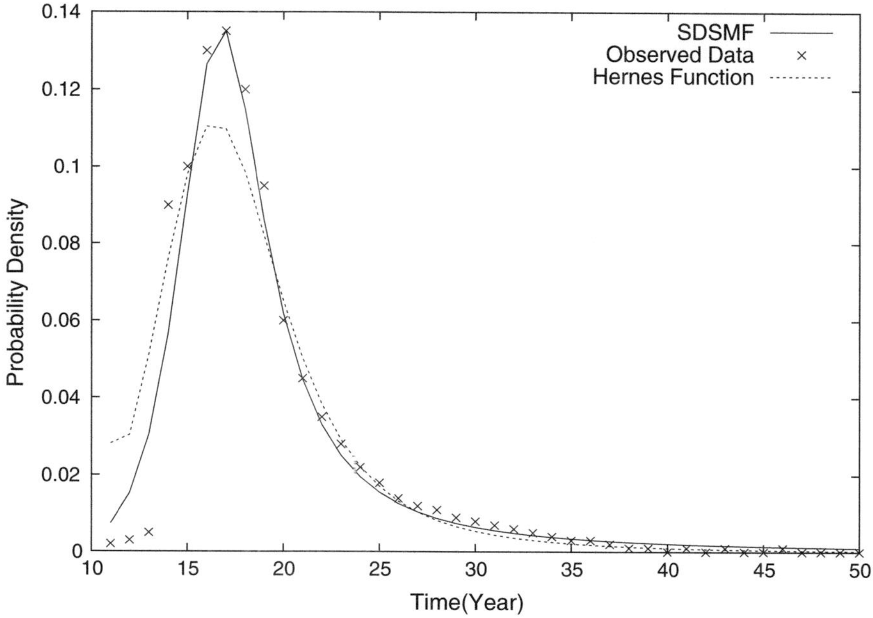

Fig. 3.7 Observed data and the application of several marriage functions for Algerian Muslims in 1948. *Source* L. Henry [28], p.57

good fit for the first half and the peak of distribution if it had been adjusted to fit the latter half. The observed data exhibits unreasonable jumps for ages 13 and 14. Although societal norms caused this jump, young marriages must exist. Only their declarations and registrations are suppressed by the married couples or by others. Applying SDSMF, we were able to estimate and interpolate more plausible values for the first half of distribution. That is to say, with SDSMF, we can more accurately calculate first marriages of those under 13 years of age, declarations of which are below their actual numbers. We suspect that the sum of undeclared marriages of those below the age of 13 years is almost equal to the difference between SDSMF and the observed value. Namely, SDSMF is robust enough for estimating true parameters, even when the data contains much noise.

3.6 Conclusion

SDSMF is the best descriptor of first marriage occurrences of females that has ever been developed. It assumes that each occurrence of first marriage is a stochastic variable. Simply put, as time t increases, stochastic values alter, depending on the ratio of those who have ever married within a residential space. This stochastic simplicity implies an absolutely significant inference that our subjective choices on whether or not to marry are trivial elements of these phenomena, because they are just the results of their surroundings and not the causes.

Marriage occurs background independently. I expect that fertility behaviors are fundamentally background independent. It is of no use to attempt to trace our consciousness to formulate the process of first marriage.

It was not until we acquired this computable marriage function that we have been able to predict fertility rates for the future.

In the world of background independence, intentions, motivations, and desires are generated *ex post facto*. Our behavior is solely the outcome of other behaviors. This reality essentially reflects background independence; a concept that will inevitably yield a rich harvest.

Appendix A
Mathematical Supplement

A.1 Transforming a Difference Equation into a Differential Equation using Taylor Expansion (one-dimensional)

Consider how $C(x, t)$ changes in the difference equation (2.3) within a very short interval of time Δt. The equation (2.3) changes within a very short interval of time Δt because of the effect of very small intervals of space Δx.

$$\begin{aligned} &c(x, t + \Delta t) \\ &= \mu\, c(x - \Delta x, t) + \mu\, c(x + \Delta x, t) + \\ &\quad (1 - 2\mu)\left[(c(x, t) + \alpha(\beta - c(x, t))(\gamma - c(x, t))\right] \end{aligned} \tag{A.1}$$

The left-hand side of the Eq. (A.1)–(2.3) is Taylor-expanded by t, and the right side by x. Both are divided by Δt. This takes into account the rate of variability.

First, the left-hand side of the Eq. (A.1) is transformed as follows. (μ is initially left out).

$$\frac{c(x, t + \Delta t) - c(x, t)}{\Delta t} = \frac{\partial c(x, t)}{\partial t}\frac{(t + \Delta t - t)}{\Delta t} + \frac{1}{2!}\frac{\partial^2 c(x, t)}{\partial t^2}\frac{(t + \Delta t - t)^2}{\Delta t} + \cdots$$

The nomials upper the second in the above equation can be ignored, because they hardly vary. After rearranging the equation, we obtain a partial differentiation (A.2):

$$\frac{c(x, t + \Delta t) - c(x, t)}{\Delta t} \doteq \frac{\partial c(x, t)}{\partial t} \tag{A.2}$$

Next, the first nomial on the right-hand side of the Eq. (A.1) is expanded as follows:

$$\frac{c(x - \Delta x, t) - c(x, t)}{\Delta x} = \frac{\partial c(x, t)}{\partial x}\frac{(x - \Delta x - x)}{\Delta t} + \frac{1}{2!}\frac{\partial^2 c(x, t)}{\partial x^2}\frac{(x - \Delta x - x)^2}{\Delta t} + \cdots$$

S. Ike, *Fertility Decline and Background Independence*,
Population Studies of Japan, DOI 10.1007/978-4-431-55151-5

The above equation is simplified as follows:

$$\frac{c(x-\Delta x,t)-c(x,t)}{\Delta x}=\frac{\partial c(x,t)}{\partial x}\frac{-\Delta x}{\Delta t}+\frac{1}{2!}\frac{\partial^2 c(x,t)}{\partial x^2}\frac{\Delta x^2}{\Delta t}+\frac{1}{3!}\frac{\partial^3 c(x,t)}{\partial x^3}\frac{-\Delta x^3}{\Delta t}+\cdots \tag{A.3}$$

Likewise, the second nomial on the right-hand side of the Eq. (A.1) is expanded as follows:

$$\frac{c(x+\Delta x,t)-c(x,t)}{\Delta x}=\frac{\partial c(x,t)}{\partial x}\frac{\Delta x}{\Delta t}+\frac{1}{2!}\frac{\partial^2 c(x,t)}{\partial x^2}\frac{\Delta x^2}{\Delta t}+\frac{1}{3!}\frac{\partial^3 c(x,t)}{\partial x^3}\frac{\Delta x^3}{\Delta t}+\cdots \tag{A.4}$$

The third nomial on the right-hand side of the Eq. (A.1) does not vary by Δx. It only varies at the space $c(x,t)$ without the effect of another space. In other words, we can consider the instantaneous variation of $c(x,t)$ based on only one variable t. The first element $c(x,t)$ of the third nomial does not change by t. We, therefore, eliminate it. The coefficient $\frac{\alpha}{\Delta t}$ remains a finite value (and even increases), because if it is ∞, then the equation is instantaneously exposed. Note that $(\beta - c(x,t))(\gamma - c(x,t))$ corresponds to the rate of variation.

The odd n-th power nomials in the Eq. (A.3) and the Eq. (A.4) canceled each other. We can ignore the nomials of the third derivatives as they are negligible. The Eq. (A.1) then transposes into the following partial differential equation:

$$\frac{\partial c(x,t)}{\partial t}=\mu\,\frac{\partial^2 c(x,t)}{\partial x^2}\frac{\Delta x^2}{\Delta t}+(1-2\mu)\frac{\alpha}{\Delta t}(\beta-c(x,t))(\gamma-c(x,t)) \tag{A.5}$$

Turning now to $\frac{\Delta x^2}{\Delta t}$, if it is infinitely small, there will be no variation of the differential equation. Therefore, we can assume that it is a finite constant. Let me express this multiplied by μ as D_1, and $(1-2\mu)\frac{\alpha}{\Delta t}$ as D_2:

$$\frac{\partial c(x,t)}{\partial t}=D_1\frac{\partial^2 c(x,t)}{\partial x^2}+D_2(\beta-c(x,t))(\gamma-c(x,t)) \tag{A.6}$$

We find a partial differential equation (A.6) similar to what is known as the logistic diffusion equation in mathematical biology. This is the **Differential Equation of the Spatial Distribution of Children (DESDC)**.

A.2 Deriving the Velocity of the Progressive Wave in Two-Dimensional Space as $\sqrt{2\mu\alpha}$

In line with R. A. Fisher's derivation of velocity in The Wave of Advance of Advantageous Genes [25] within one-dimensional space, we postulate that the progressive wave maintains a fixed shape. Kametaka [32] gave a proof for this fixed shape of the progressive wave. That is, the front (edge) of the wave maintains a constant velocity v. Based on this postulation, we can express the following partial difference equation:

$$\frac{\partial c}{\partial t} = v\left(\frac{\partial c}{\partial x} + \frac{\partial c}{\partial y}\right) \tag{A.7}$$

We can express the following reaction-diffusion equation that does not involve t:

$$\mu\left(\frac{\partial^2 c}{\partial x^2} + \frac{\partial^2 c}{\partial x^2}\right) - v\left(\frac{\partial c}{\partial x} + \frac{\partial c}{\partial y}\right) + \alpha(\beta - c)(\gamma - c) = 0 \tag{A.8}$$

The parameters of space x, y are expressed using the gradient of the mean number of children in space as follows g, h:

$$g = \frac{\partial c}{\partial x}, \qquad h = \frac{\partial c}{\partial y}$$

Hence we can express the following two equations:

$$\frac{\partial^2 c}{\partial x^2} = \frac{\partial g}{\partial x} = g\frac{\partial g}{\partial c} \tag{A.9}$$

$$\frac{\partial^2 c}{\partial y^2} = \frac{\partial h}{\partial y} = h\frac{\partial h}{\partial c} \tag{A.10}$$

We now arrive at the following equation:

$$\mu\left(g\frac{\partial g}{\partial c} + h\frac{\partial h}{\partial c}\right) + v(g + h) + \alpha(\beta - c)(\gamma - c) = 0 \tag{A.11}$$

The front (edge) of the progressive wave is also the inflection point of the mean number of children. So $\frac{\partial^2 c}{\partial x^2}$ is 0 implies $\frac{\partial g}{\partial c}$ is 0. Likewise, $\frac{\partial h}{\partial c}$ is also 0, and $v(g + h) = -\alpha(\beta - c)(\gamma - c)$.

This inflection point creates the gradient through the effect of the reaction nomial. As a result of this gradient, c declines in a chain reaction. Thus, the front of the wave advances.

When β approaches c, g/c, h/c approaches certain limits, u, z, that is, the minimum of the mean number of the children. Therefore, u, z must satisfy the following equality . In this case, we can select a constant for $(\beta - c)(\gamma - c)$, depending on the selection of β' when it is asymptotically approaching β.

$$\mu(u^2 + z^2) + v(u + z) + \alpha = 0 \tag{A.12}$$

As we assume the isotropy of space, $u = z$.

$$2\mu u^2 + 2vu + \alpha = 0 \tag{A.13}$$

Hence, we express the above quadratic equation. The value u must be a real number, because u is the quantum of the decline in the mean number of children. Therefore, a quadratic equation in u, which has a real root, is only possible if the following discriminant is greater than 0.

$$(2v)^2 - 4 \times 2\mu\alpha \geq 0 \tag{A.14}$$

We arrange this as:

$$v \geq \sqrt{2\mu\alpha} \tag{A.15}$$

We now obtain the velocity of the progressive wave in two-dimensional space as $\sqrt{2\mu\alpha}$. The combined transformation of $\sqrt{2\mu\alpha}$ is $2\sqrt{\mu\alpha}$, which is the velocity in one- dimensional space.

References

1. Beaver, M.W. 1973. Population, infant mortality and milk. *Population Studies*, 27(2): 243–254.
2. Becker, Gray S. 1978. *The economic approach to human behavior*. Chicago: The University of Chicago Press.
3. Becker, Gray S. 1981. *A treatise on the family*. Cambridge: Harvard University Press.
4. Caldwell, John Charles. 1982. *Population and social structure: Theory of fertility decline*. London: Academic Press.
5. Calot, Gérard. 1998. *Two centuries of Swiss demographic history–Graphic album of the 1860–2050 period*. Swiss Federal Statistical Office/Observatoire démographque européen, Paris. with assistance from Alan Confession and Jean-Paul Sardon(Observatoire démographque européen, Paris). Erminio Baranzini, Stephane Cotter and Philippe Wanner(Swiss Federal Statistical Office), ISBN 3-303-01095-1.
6. Carlsson, G. 1966. The decline of fertility: Innovation or adjustment process. *Population Studies* 20(2): 149–174.
7. Cigno, Alessandro. 1991. *Economics of the family*. Oxford: Oxford University Press.
8. Cleland, John and Wilson, Christopher. 1987. Demand theories of the fertility transition:An iconoclastic view. *Population Studies*, (41):5–30.
9. Coale, A.J., and D.R. McNeil. 1972. The distribution by age of the frequency of first marriage in a female cohort. *Journal of the American Statistical Association* 67(340): 743–749.
10. Coale, Ansley J. 1967. Factors associated with the development of low fertility: An historic summary, in united nations. In *Proceedings of the World Population Conference, Belgrade*, Vol. 2, New York, United Nations.
11. Coale, Ansley J. 1971. Age patterns of marriage. *Population Studies* 25(2): 193–214.
12. Coale, Ansley J. 1973. The demographic transition. In *IUSSP International Conference*, Liège. vol 1, 53–72.
13. Coale, A.J., and Treadway, R. 1986. A summary of the changing distribution of overall fertility, marital fertility, and the proportion married in provinces of Europe. In: *The Decline of Fertility in Europe—The Revised Proceedings of a Conference on the Princeton European Fertility Project*—eds. Ansley J.Coale and Susan Cotts Watkins, Princeton. Conference on the Princeton European Fertility Project (1979), Princeton University Press.
14. Coale, Ansley J., and T.J. Trussell. 1974. Model fertility schedules: Variations in the age structure of childbearing in human population. *Population Index* 40: 185–258.
15. Coale, Ansley J., and Watkins, Susan Cotts. 1986. The decline of fertility in Europe since the eighteenth century as a chapter in human demographic history. In: *The Decline of Fertility in Europe—The Revised Proceedings of a Conference on the Princeton European Fertility Project*— eds. Ansley J. Coale and Susan Cotts Watkins, Princeton. Conference on the Princeton European Fertility Project (1979), Princeton University Press.

S. Ike, *Fertility Decline and Background Independence*,
Population Studies of Japan, DOI 10.1007/978-4-431-55151-5

16. Conlisk, John, Gong, Jyh-Chyi, and Ching. H. Tong. 2000. Dynamics of imitation. *Journal of Mathematical Sociology* 24(2): 97–128.
17. Dawkins, Richard. 1989. *The selfish gene*. Oxford: Oxford University Press.
18. Dennis, J.E. Jr., and Daniel J. Woods. 1985. Optimization on microcomputers the nelder-mead simplex algorithm. Technical report, Rice University, available as Math. Science TR 85-9.
19. Easterlin, R.A. 1961. The American baby boom in historical perspective. *American Economic Review* 51(5): 869–911.
20. Easterlin, R.A. 1968. *Population laborforce and long swing in economic growth: The American experience*. New york: Columbia University Press.
21. Easterlin, R.A. 1987. *Birth and fortune: The impact of numbers on personal welfare*. Chicago: The University of Chicago Press.
22. Ehmer, Josef. 2004. *Bevölkerungsgeshichite und historishe Demographie 1800–2000*. Múnchen: Oldenbourg Wissenshaftsverlag GmbH.
23. Feller, William. 1957. *An introduction to probability theory and its applications*. 2nd ed. New York: Wiley.
24. Patrick, Festy. 1984. *Fertility in Western Countries from 1870 to 1970*. Population Studies Translation Series No.7. The Population Devision Economic and Social Commission for Asia and the Pacific. United Nations, Bangkok.
25. Fisher, R.A. 1937. The wave of advance of advantageous genes. *Ann Eugen* 7: 355–369.
26. Habakkuk, H.J. 1965. English population in the eighteen century. In *Population in History*, ed. Glass and Eversley. London: Edward Arnold.
27. Henkel, Ramon E. 1979. Tests of significance. *Quantitative Applications in the Social Sciences*. Beverly Hills/London: SAGE.
28. Henry, Louis. 1976. *Population: Analysis and models*. London: Edward Arnold. *Démographie:analysis et modèles* (trans: Etienne van de Walle and Elise F. Jones).
29. Hernes, Gudmund. 1972. The process of entry into first marriage. *Americal Sociological Review* 37: 173–182.
30. Ike, Shuichirou. 2012. A singularity of fertility decline is Lot-et-Garonne. *Journal of Mathematical Sociology* 36: 137–155. doi:10.1080/0022250X.2011.556917.
31. Ike, Shuuichirou. 2002. A non-stationary stochastic process model of completed marital fertility. *Journal of Mathematical Sociology* 26: 35–55.
32. Kametaka, Koremichi. 1977. *Hi-senkei Bibun Houteishiki*, volume 19 of *Surikaiseki to sono Shuuhen*. Sangyoutosho Kabusikigaisya.
33. Kawabe, Hiroshi. 1981. The educational developement and fertility in the pre-war Japan. *Journal of Population Problems(Jinko Mondai Kenkyu)* (158): 1–10.
34. Kerlin, Samuel. 1971. *A first course in stochastic processes*. 4th edn. San Diego: Academic Press.
35. Keyfitz, Nathan. 1977. *Applied mathematical demography*, 2nd edn. Berlin: Springer.
36. Knodel, John, and Etienne van de Walle. 1979. Lessons from the past: Policy implications of historical fertility studies. *Populations and Development Review* 5: 217–245.
37. Knodel, John E. 1977. Family limitation and the fertility transition: Evidence from the age patterns of fertility in Europe and Asia. *Population Studies* 31(2): 219–249.
38. Knodel, John E. 1988. *Demographic behavior in the past: A study of fourteen German village populations in the eighteenth and nineteenth centuries*. Cambridge studies in population, economy and society in past time 6. Cambridge: Cambridge University Press.
39. Knodel, John E., Aphichat Chamratrithirong, and Nibhon Debavalya. 1987. *Thailand's reproductive revolution: Rapid fertility decline in a Third-world setting*. Social Demography. Madison: University of Wisconsin Press.
40. Kohler, H.P. 1997. Learning in social networks and contraceptive choice. *Demography* 34(3): 369–383.
41. Kolmogorov, A.N. 1931. Über die Analitischen Methoden Wahrscheinlichkeitsrechnung. *Mathematische Annalen* 104: 415–458.
42. Kolmogorov, A.N. 1933. *Grundbeguriffe der Wahrscheinlichkeitsrechnung*. Berlin: Springer.

43. Kolmogroff, A., I. Petrovsky, and N. Piscounoff. 1937. étude de l'equation de la diffusion avec croissance de la quantité de matière et son application à un problème bibliogique. *Bull. Univ. d'État à Moscou*, Ser, Internat. Sect.A:1–25.
44. Mayer, K.U. and N.B.Tuma. 1990. *Event history analysis in life course research*. Madison: The University of Wisconsin Press
45. Naikaku Toukei Kyoku. *Kokusei Tyousa Igo Nihon Jinkou Toukei Shusei*, volume Taisyou Shouwa Senzenhen(Before WWII) 2,3,4,5. Touyou Syorin, 1994. Nihon Teikoku Jinkou Doutai Toukei no Huxtukokuban. Published: Hara Shobou.
46. Levine, D. 1977. *Family formation in an age of nascent capitalism*. San Diego: Academic Press, Inc.
47. Libet, Benjamin. 2004. *MIND TIME—The temporal factor in consciousness*. Cambridge: Harvard University Press.
48. Marchetti, Cesare, Perrin S. Meyer, and Jesse H. Ausubel. 1996. Human population dynamics revisited with the logistic model: How much can be modeled and predicted? *Technological Forecasting and Social Change* 52: 1–30.
49. McKeown, T., R.G. Brown, and R G. Recode. 1972. An interpretation of the modern rise of population in Europe. *Populstion Studies* 26(3): 345–382.
50. McKeown, Thomas. 1978. Fertility, mortality and causes of death. *Population Studies* 32(3): 535–542.
51. McKeown, Thomas, R.G. Recoed, and R.D. Turner. 1975. An interpretation of the decline of mortarity in England and Wales during the twentieth century. *Population Studies* 29(3): 391–422.
52. McKeown, Thomas, and R.G. Record. 1962. Reasons for the Decline of mortality in England and Wales during the nineteen century. *Population Studies* 16(2): 94–122.
53. Ministry of Internal Affairs Statistics Bureau of Japan and Communications. 1973. *Sangyou betu Syugyousya no Jikeiretu Hikaku(Taishou 9 nen Kokuseityousa— Shouwa 45 nen Kokuseityousa*. Number 3 in Shouwa 45 nen Kokuseityousa series. Tokyo: Japan Statistical Association.
54. Montgomery, M.R., and J.B. Casterline. 1993. The diffusion of fertility control in Taiwan: Evidence from pooled cross-section time-series models. *Population Studies* 47(3): 457–479.
55. Montgomery, M.R., and J.B. Casterline. 1996. Social learning, social influence, and new models of fertility. *Population and Development Review* 22(Supplement): 151–175.
56. Nemhauser, G.L., A.H.G. Rinnooy Kan, and M.J.Todd, eds. 1989. *Optimization*, Vol. 1. *Handbooks in Operations Research and Management Science*. Amsterdam: Elsevier Science Publishers.
57. Nørretranders, Tor. 1998. *The user illusion: Cutting consciousness down to size*, illustrated edn. New York: Viking Adult (April 1, 1998).
58. Notestein, Frank. W. 1945. Population–the long view. In *Food for the world*, ed. Theodore W. Shultz, 36–57. Chicago: University of Chicago Press.
59. Rosero-Bixby, L., and J.B. Casterline. 1993. Modeling diffusion effects in fertility transition. *Population Studies* 47(1): 147–167
60. Sharin, Allan. 1986. Urban-rural differences in fertility in Europe during the deographic transition. In *The Decline of Fertility in Europe—The Revised Proceedings of a Conference on the Princeton European Ferility Project—*, eds. Ansley J. Coale and Susan Cotts Watkins, Princeton. Conference on the Princeton European Fertility Project (1979), Princeton University Press.
61. Skellam, J.G. 1951. Random dispersal in theoretical populations. *Biometrika* 38: 196–218.
62. Sourihu Toukei Kyouku. 1953. *Showa 35 nen Kokuseityousa Houkoku Dai 4 kan Todouhukenhen*. Ookura shou Insatukyoku.
63. Stolnitz, George J. 1964. The demographic transition: From height to low birth rates and death rates. In *Population: The vital revolution*, ed. R.Freedman, Chapter 2, 30–46. New York: Doubleday.
64. Teitelbaum, M.S., and J.M. Winter. 1985. *The fear of population decline*. San Diego: Academic Press.
65. Turing, Alan Mathison. 1952. The chemical basis of morphogenesis. *Philosophical Transactions of The Royal Society of London* 237: 37–72.

66. van de Walle, Etienne, and John Knodel. 1967. Demographic transition and fertility decline: The European case. In *the International Union for the Scientific Study of Population*, 47–55. Sidney Conference.
67. Woods, Daniel J. 1985. *An interactive approach for solving multi-objective optimization problems*. Ph.D thesis, Rice University, available as Math. Science TR 85-5.

Index

S. Ike, *Fertility Decline and Background Independence*,
Population Studies of Japan, DOI 10.1007/978-4-431-55151-5

MIX
Papier aus verantwortungsvollen Quellen
Paper from responsible sources
FSC® C105338
FSC
www.fsc.org

If you have any concerns about our products,
you can contact us on
ProductSafety@springernature.com

In case Publisher is established outside the EU,
the EU authorized representative is:
Springer Nature Customer Service Center GmbH
Europaplatz 3, 69115 Heidelberg, Germany

Printed by Libri Plureos GmbH
in Hamburg, Germany